Health-Related Fitness
for Grades 3 and 4

Chris Hopper, PhD
Humboldt State University

Bruce Fisher
Fortuna Elementary School

Kathy D. Munoz, EdD
Humboldt State University

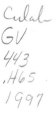

Human Kinetics

We dedicate this book to our families—

Renee, Molly, Ian, and Andrew;

Rich, Heather, Wesley, and Ryan;

Mindi and Jenny.

Library of Congress Cataloging-in-Publication Data

Hopper, Christopher A., 1952–
    Health-related fitness for grades 3 and 4 / Chris Hopper, Kathy Munoz,
Bruce Fisher.
        p.   cm.
    Includes index.
    ISBN 0-87322-499-X
    1. Physical fitness for children.   2. Health education
(Elementary)   3. Cardiovascular system—Diseases—Prevention.
I. Munoz, Kathy, 1951– .II. Fisher, Bruce, 1949– .
III. Title.
GV443.H65   1997
361.7'042—dc20   96-11314
                                                   CIP

ISBN: 0-87322-499-X

Acquisitions Editor: Scott Wikgren; **Developmental Editor:** Nanette Smith; **Assistant Editor:** Henry Woolsey; **Editorial Assistant:** Coree Schutter; **Copyeditors:** Denelle Eknes, Julia Anderson; **Indexer:** Barbara E. Cohen; **Typesetting and Layout:** Impressions Book and Journal Services, Inc.; **Graphic Designer:** Judy Henderson; **Cover Designer:** Jack Davis; **Illustrators:** Mary Yemma Long, Nicole Barbuto, Craig Ronto, Dianna Porter; **Printer:** Versa Press

Printed in the United States of America

10 9 8 7 6 5 4 3 2 1

Human Kinetics
Web site: http://www.humankinetics.com/

United States: Human Kinetics
P.O. Box 5076, Champaign, IL 61825-5076
1-800-747-4457
e-mail: humank@hkusa.com

Canada: Human Kinetics
Box 24040, Windsor, ON N8Y 4Y9
1-800-465-7301 (in Canada only)
e-mail: humank@hkcanada.com

Europe: Human Kinetics
P.O. Box IW14, Leeds LS16 6TR, United Kingdom
(44) 1132 781708
e-mail: humank@hkeurope.com

Australia: Human Kinetics
57A Price Avenue, Lower Mitcham, South Australia 5062
(08) 277 1555
e-mail: humank@hkaustralia.com

New Zealand: Human Kinetics
P.O. Box 105-231, Auckland 1
(09) 523 3462
e-mail: humank@hknewz.com

Contents

Preface

In recent years the following headlines have appeared in the media:

Young Adults More Fat Than Fit, Study Finds

Lorem ipsum dolor sit amet, consectetuer adipiscing elit, euismod tinci magna aliquam enim ad minim erci tation ulla nisl ut aliquip e Duis autem vel drerit in vulput sequat, vel illu facilisis at vero

Lorem ipsum dolor sit amet, consectetuer

Young People's Health Declining, Report Says

Lorem ipsum dolor sit amet, consectetuer adipiscing elit, sed diam nonummy nibh euismod tincidunt ut laoreet dolore magna aliquam erat volutpat. Ut wisi enim ad minim veniam, quis nostrud exerci tation ullamcorper suscipit lobortis nisl ut aliquip ex ea commodo consequat. Duis autem vel eum iriure dolor in hendrerit in vulputate velit esse molestie consequat, vel illum dolore eu feugi accumsan et iusto odio dignissim qui b delenit augue duis dolore te feugait nulla amet, consectetuer adipiscing elit, sed tincidunt ut laoreet dolore magna aliqua ad minim veniam, quis nostrud exerci ta tis nisl ut aliquip ex ea commodo conseq Duis autem vel eum iriure dolor in hend lestie consequat, vel illum dolore eu feug accumsan et iusto odio dignissim qui b delenit augue duis dolore te feugait nulla soluta nobis eleifend option congue ni mazim placerat facer possim assum.

FITNESS: Study Finds Big Slip

Lorem ipsum dolor sit amet, consectetuer adipiscing elit, sed diam nonummy nibh euismod tincidunt ut laoreet dolore

lore te feugait nulla facilisi. tempor cum soluta nobis elei congue nihil imperdiet domi erat facer possim a m dolor sit amet, elit, sed diam non tincidunt ut lao quam e nim ve ullamc ip ex e vel eu lputate vero ero

Vigorous Exercise Adds On Years, Study Says

Lorem ipsum dolor sit amet, consectetuer adipiscing elit, sed diam nonummy nibh euismod tincidunt ut laoreet dolore magna aliquam erat volutpat. Ut wisi enim ad minim veniam, quis nostrud ex erci tation ullamcorper suscipit lobortis nisl ut aliquip ex ea commodo consequat. Duis autem vel eum iriure dolor in hendrerit in vulputate velit esse molestie con

sequat, vel illum dolore eu feugiat nulla facilisis at vero eros et accumsan et iusto odio dignissim qui blandit praesent lupta tum zzril delenit augue duis dolore te feu gait nulla facilisi. Lorem ipsum dolor sit amet, consectetuer adipiscing elit, sed diam nonummy nibh euismod tincidunt ut laoreet dolore magna aliquam erat vo lutpat. Ut wisi enim ad minim veniam,

Any Exercise is Good Exercise: Experts say even a little moderate activity goes a long way

Lorem ipsum dolor sit amet, consectetuer adipiscing elit, sed diam nonummy nibh eu ismod tincidunt ut laoreet dolore magna ali volutpat. Ut wisi enim ad minim uis nostrud exerci tation ullamcor bit lobortis nisl ut aliquip ex ea consequat. Duis autem vel eum or in hendrerit in vulputate velit

Lorem ipsum dolor sit amet, consectetuer adipiscing elit, sed diam nonummy nibh eu ismod tincidunt ut laoreet dolore magna ali quam erat volutpat. Ut wisi enim ad minim veniam, quis nostrud exerci tation ullamcor per suscipit lobortis nisl ut aliquip ex ea commodo consequat. Duis autem vel eum iriure dolor in hendrerit in vulputate velit

Kids Confused On Health, Survey Finds

Lorem ipsum dolor sit amet, consectetuer

facilisis at vero eros et accumsan et iusto lupta e feu r cum t. nihil plac

FAT: Even Moderate Weight Gains Are Risky

Lorem ipsum dolor sit amet, consectetuer

amet, consectetuer adipiscing elit, sed m nonummy nibh euismod tincidunt aoreet dolore magna aliquam erat vo Ut wisi enim ad minim veniam, nostrud exerci tation ullamcorper cipit lobortis nisl ut aliquip ex ea com lo consequat. s autem vel eum iriure dolor in hen rit in vulputate velit esse molestie con quat, vel illum dolore eu feugiat nulla lisis at vero eros et accumsan et iusto o dignissim qui blandit praesent lupta zzril delenit augue duis dolore te feu nulla facilisi. Nam liber tempor cum

tetuer nibh dolore d wisi d ex bortis quat. hen te con nulla iusto lupta te feu lor sit , sed idunt at vo

Overall, considerable evidence suggests that the cardiovascular health of children is at risk.

As a teacher, you're as concerned about the cardiovascular health of kids as are parents and medical professionals. You know if kids develop healthy habits when they're in elementary school, chances are they'll become healthy adolescents and adults. With the lively and seasoned activities and lessons in this book, you can incorporate sound cardiovascular wellness into your classroom. Whether you are an elementary school teacher developing physical education lessons or a physical education specialist, you'll find this an invaluable and complete guide to promoting cardiovascular health through daily lessons.

Chris Hopper and Kathy Munoz teach in the Department of Health and Physical Education at Humboldt State University and have worked extensively with teachers in Northern California to improve the instruction in physical education and nutrition. Their work has been published in research journals such as Research Quarterly for Exercise and Sport and teacher journals such as Learning. Bruce Fisher was California Teacher of the Year in 1991 and serves as a consultant for health education to the California Department of Education. Bruce is recognized by his colleagues as an innovative teacher. All three authors have tested the lessons in this book, which represents a decade of professional work.

The authors designed this book to enhance existing physical education programs and to be a comprehensive resource for teachers who want to spice up their teaching with fun-filled, exciting learning activities. This book includes physical education activity lessons that emphasize children enjoying movement.

The fitness and nutrition information includes cardiovascular fitness, strength, endurance, flexibility, fat, carbohydrates, water, sodium, and heart-healthy eating. The goal of the book is to communicate the need for a lifelong commitment to health and physical fitness, using cardiovascular exercise and diet. The goal for you in using the book is to change the attitudes and behaviors of children so they embrace this commitment to health and fitness. The book emphasizes ready-to-go activities and materials teachers can easily use. The book has a user friendly approach with illustrations, pages to copy, and lesson outlines. We recognize that classroom teachers are extremely busy. The format and design eliminate extra work.

Teachers can meet multiple teaching objectives by using this curriculum. Unique features include across-the-curriculum activities, meaningful homework, and cooperative learning activities. In addition, while children are studying fitness and nutrition, they'll be developing research techniques (surveys), critical thinking skills (comparing foods), science concepts (e.g., how the heart works), language arts (e.g., food label analysis), and mathematical applications (e.g., counting pulse rates).

The program covers nine weeks of fitness and nutrition education and activities related to cardiovascular health. Each week includes five 30-minute lessons, with one concept development and discussion lesson, three physical education activity lessons, and one nutrition concept lesson. The lessons are divided into the following sections:

Heart Facts (1 week)

What's in a Workout? (1 week)

Fitness Components (1 week)

Risk Factors (1 week)

Aerobic Fitness concepts (2 weeks)

Flexibility Fitness concepts (1 week)

Strength Fitness concepts (1 week)

Healthy Lifestyle (1 week)

This book is the second in a series of three books designed to enhance the cardiovascular health of children. Be sure to review *Health-Related Fitness for Grades 1 and 2* and *Health-Related Fitness for Grades 5 and 6.*

Acknowledgments

We thank the following teachers for help in pilot testing: Linda Provancha, Fred Johansen, Steve Wartburg, and Linda Buron.

We also thank Tami Jaegel for researching information, and Ira Samuels and Mike Mullane for their advice.

We thank Tricia Gill, Elissa Fisher, and Linda Baxter for typing the manuscript.

Introduction to Curriculum

Before starting the curriculum, include an introduction to the lessons and explain the lesson objectives and purposes.

Objectives

1. To teach the basic elements of a healthy cardiovascular system (lungs, heart, and blood vessels)
2. To introduce important fitness and nutrition concepts for a healthy heart
3. To teach children how to plan and develop their own exercise programs

Teaching Strategies

- Use laminated task cards with names of specific exercises and activities that you can use as a resource. Use the exercises in chapter 13 to develop cards.
- Stress that children don't have heart attacks. Children develop lifestyle habits that put them at risk for heart disease later in life.
- Avoid simply repeating jumping jacks, windmills, and so forth, with no purpose. Put them into a game or activity.
- Don't use running laps or other exercises as a punishment for bad behavior.
- Use writing projects about exercise and nutrition to improve language arts.
- Avoid elimination activities.

Cross-Curricular Themes

We have identified the following cross-curricular areas in the lessons:

- Health

- Visual and Performing Arts

- Science

- Mathematics

- Language Arts

Nutrition Education

In nutrition education students gain the knowledge, skills, and motivation they need to make wise food choices. They learn that healthy foods are intimately connected with physical, mental, emotional, and social health. Also, energy, self-image, and physical fitness are related to heart-healthy nutrition. A comprehensive nutrition education program integrates nutrition lessons with the core curriculum. Lessons in this book include classroom activities for food tasting, preparation, and menu planning.

Home Activities

Home activities provide a connection between the home and the school, strengthening the school-family relationship. Parents as care providers can dramatically influence eating habits and physical activity levels. They buy and prepare food for children and determine restaurant choices. In addition, parents help their children make significant choices regarding exercise. Parents can register their children for sport and activity programs and tell their children to turn off the television. In overall lifestyle, parents serve as gatekeepers, and children are unlikely to change their lifestyles without the support of their parents.

A Lesson a Day for Nine Weeks

We organized the curriculum to provide a lesson a day for nine weeks. This concentrated approach will give students the knowledge and skills to make significant lifestyle changes. The curriculum is sequential, with basic knowledge introduced, then applied to cardiovascular health.

Discussion Lessons

Discussion lessons are an essential component of the curriculum and allow students to reflect on important concepts about physical fitness and nutrition. These lessons develop the skills and knowledge of physical fitness and nutrition that are the foundation of a healthy lifestyle.

Warming Up and Cooling Down

Each lesson should start with a warm-up and finish with a cool-down.

Warm-Up = Light Activity + Stretching

A warm-up before exercise prepares your body for activity and avoids "jump starting" the body. Warm-ups stretch muscles and help prevent muscle soreness and injury. In addition, warm-ups prepare the heart for more vigorous activity and avoid adding stress.

Exercise specialists recommend completing light activity first, such as jogging, followed by gentle static stretching (see basic warm-up and cool-down stretches). Remember not to bounce when stretching. A listing of warm-up activities is found on page 101. Most of these include jogging or light running.

Although children rarely stretch before going out to recess or playing vigorous activities, stretching is an investment for the future. Joints that are flexible in childhood will gradually lose mobility with age, leading to a reduced range of movement. Developing a lifetime habit of stretching before exercise can pay dividends now and later.

Cool-Down = Less Vigorous Activity + Stretching

The cool-down is an essential part of any exercise session. It is just as important as the warm-up. A cool-down should last about five minutes and allow your body to gently recover after vigorous exercise. An abrupt end to exercise sends your blood pressure fluctuating like a yo-yo. This leads to slow removal of waste products. Light activity and stretching continue the pumping action of muscles on veins, helping the circulation remove wastes. Static stretching may help reduce delayed soreness or muscle pain the day after exercise. Cool-down activities are found on page 103.

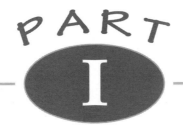

Weekly Lessons

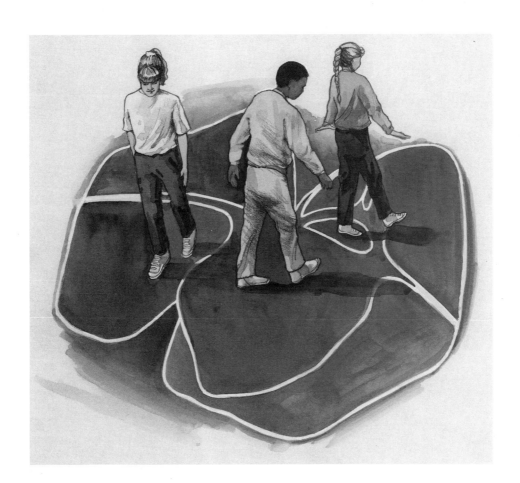

Week 1: Heart Facts

The lessons emphasize key functions of the heart and the circulatory system in the first week. The nutrition information introduces the distinction between animal and plant fats.

WEEK 1

Lesson 1

Body Beats

Goals

- To learn that a heartbeat represents the pumping action of the heart
- To learn individual heart rate

Key Concepts

Heart rates can vary between children. Most elementary school children have a pulse rate of 75 to 95 beats per minute. Generally, a boy's pulse rate is lower than a girl's. A lower rate indicates a more effective cardiovascular system.

Materials

1. Stethoscope or paper towel tube
2. Turkey baster
3. Alcohol wipes (optional)

Activity: Body Beats

Pair students by gender. To hear the pumping action of the heart, use a stethoscope or paper towel tube. The sound "lub-dub" can be heard. To allow each student to hear the heartbeat, press one end of a cardboard tube against a partner's chest. Put your ear to the other end and listen to the constant rhythm—lub-dub. Count the heart rate. Every lub-dub equals one beat. Girls and boys should have a heart rate of about 80 beats per minute. To demonstrate the pumping action of the heart, use a turkey baster. Explain that the heart is a muscle and muscle contractions force blood out of the heart to the body. If students are unable to hear a beat, have them complete some exercises to raise their heart rate. Students can open and close a hand to demonstrate pumping action of the heart until fatigue sets in. Note that the heart keeps beating continuously, but opening and closing a hand results in fatigue. Therefore, the heart muscle has to be very strong.

Teaching Tips

Use a model heart to show children the structure of the heart. Invite the school nurse into the classroom to demonstrate the use of the stethoscope. Stethoscopes may be available from American Heart Association kits. Use alcohol wipes to clean ear pieces after each use. Put one hand up in the air for one minute and then hold down for one minute. Examine the color of the hand. Discuss circulation and gravity. What would happen during zero gravity? What would happen during space travel in zero gravity? Most astronauts' faces appear puffy because of changes in the circulatory system.

WEEK 1

Lesson 2

Chamber Circuit

Goals

- To understand that blood travels between the lungs and the heart
- To improve cardiovascular endurance

Key Concepts

Teach the flow of blood through the heart (see fig. 1.1). Blood leaves the heart from the left ventricle to supply the body with oxygen. After giving up oxygen, blood returns to the heart, entering the right auricle, and is pumped into the right ventricle before going to the lungs to receive fresh oxygen. Blood with a fresh supply of oxygen returns to the left auricle and passes into the left ventricle. This lesson expands the concept of four chambers by introducing the flow of blood from the heart to the body.

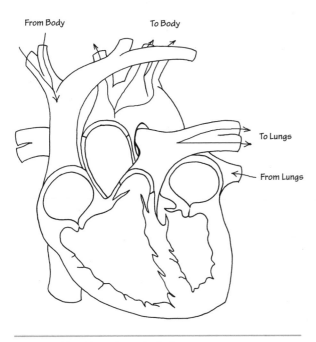

From Body   To Body

To Lungs

From Lungs

Fig. 1.1. Blood flow through the heart

Materials

1. Playground chalk, jump ropes, cones, or other markers
2. Basketballs or soccer balls (optional)
3. Cards—To lungs, From lungs, To body, From body

Warm-Up: 5 Minutes

Select stretching and warm-up activities.

Activity: Chamber Circuit

- In the gym, or on the playground or field, mark an outline (at least the size of a basketball court) using chalk, jump ropes, or cones including the heart, lungs, head, feet, and arms (see fig. 1.2).

- Have students follow the flow of blood through the heart, and to the body and lungs.
- Label with cards the exit and entry areas of the heart (e.g., to body, to lungs).
- Show students the blood flow pattern, then divide them into groups with a rotating leader. Make sure the first leader knows the pattern, and if necessary take all first leaders through the pattern.
- Students follow the leader through the chambers and jog to the body and lungs following the circuit of blood. Groups of students can visit all parts of the body before changing leaders. Ensure new leaders are familiar with the route.
- After students learn the blood flow, tell them to skip sideways through the valves in the heart because the pathway is narrower through these one-way valves.

Cool-Down: 5 Minutes

Select stretching and cool-down activities.

Teaching Tips

Vary the form of movement to practice—skipping, hopping, galloping, leaping, and running sideways. If you do the lesson outside, you can increase the distance. Emphasize that blood does not stand still and is always moving. Describing the blood-flow pattern in the classroom before the lesson is essential. Use fig. 1.2 in class to describe the route the leaders will take. Students can dribble basketballs or soccer balls as they move through the circuit as an extra activity, or a few children can dribble a ball and trade off to others. Students may get confused with right and left sides of the heart. They can put the diagram on their chest to determine right from left. Children with physical disabilities can move at their own speed and be a group leader.

WEEK 1

Lesson 3

Veins and Arteries

Goals

- To reinforce the pattern of blood flow
- To learn the functions of veins and arteries

Key Concepts

Blood transports oxygen to the body through the arteries. Blood without oxygen, which carries carbon

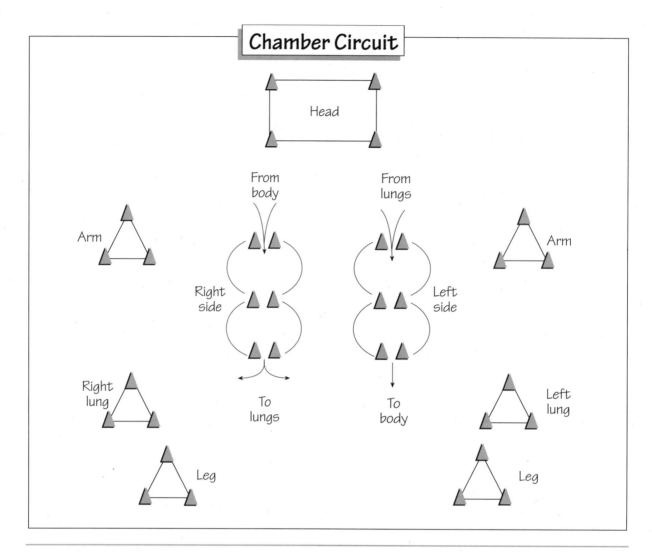

Fig. 1.2. *Chamber circuit*

dioxide, returns to the heart in the veins. The heart pumps oxygenated blood to the muscle cells to provide the energy to do work. During exercise the body needs a constant supply of oxygen.

Materials

1. Playground chalk, jump ropes, or other markers
2. Bean bags (preferably red and blue) or color-coded Popsicle sticks
3. Bean bag containers or boxes (seven)
4. Nerf balls for taggers

Warm-Up: 5 Minutes

Select stretching and warm-up activities.

Activity: Veins and Arteries

- Mark out with playground chalk, jump ropes, or cones areas representing the heart, lungs, head, arms, and legs (see fig. 1.3)
- Starting in the heart, trace the flow of blood from the heart by running to a body part.
- The students take a red bean bag (or Popsicle stick) with them to represent a molecule of oxygen and leave it at the body part in a box.
- The students move back to the heart carrying a molecule of carbon dioxide (blue bean bag).
- Every time a student comes back to the heart, they should go to the lungs to release the carbon dioxide, drop the blue bean bag, and pick up a red bean bag. They return to the heart before making a trip to another body part.

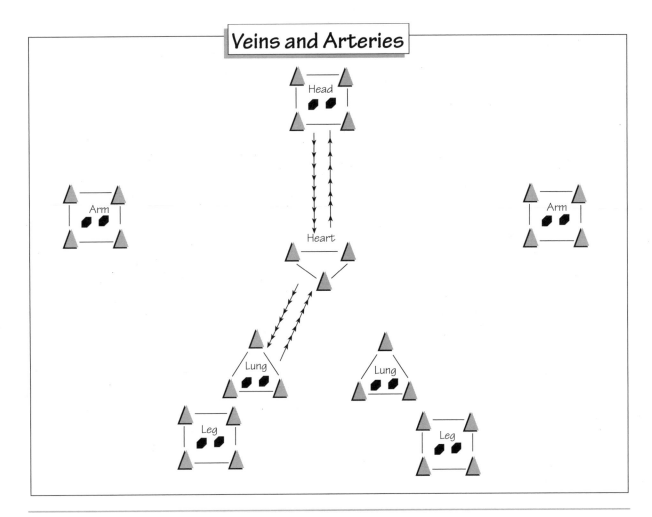

Fig. 1.3. *Veins and arteries*

- After children have learned the movement pattern, reinforce the function of arteries and veins.
- Start students in the heart, and on the command "Arteries," the students move away from the heart to a different part of the body.
- Students wait in the body periphery, and on the command "Veins," the students move back to the heart. Introduce the concept of moving faster (run or jog) in the arteries and slower (jog or walk) in the veins.

Cool-Down: 5 Minutes

Select stretching and cool-down activities.

Teaching Tips

This can also be a tag game. Have one person be "it." The teacher says "Arteries" and the students must run away from the heart. The head, arms, and feet are safe areas. When the teacher says "Veins," students return to the heart via the lungs, which are also safe areas. Tagged students become taggers. Play until everyone is tagged.

Emphasize efficient running techniques:

- Use arms by swinging forward and backward with elbows bent.
- Keep head still and upright.
- Heel hits ground first.
- Legs and feet swing and land straight ahead.

WEEK 1

Lesson 4

Oxygen Grab

Goals

- To understand the concept that muscles need oxygen to work effectively
- To improve cardiovascular endurance

Key Concepts

Muscles and bones working together allow body parts to move. Muscles need oxygen to complete movements. Explain that oxygen consists of molecules, although these molecules cannot be seen.

Materials

1. Five balloons
2. Thirty small Nerf balls or tennis balls
3. Cones
4. Two boxes labeled heart and muscle

Warm-Up: 5 Minutes

Select stretching and warm-up activities.

Activity: Oxygen Grab

- Mark out an area in the shape of a muscle (see fig. 1.4) with cones.
- Place five students acting as muscle cells inside the muscle with a balloon.
- Hand out one ball to each of the remaining students, who stand on either side of the muscle. These students act as blood cells with oxygen molecules (Nerf balls).

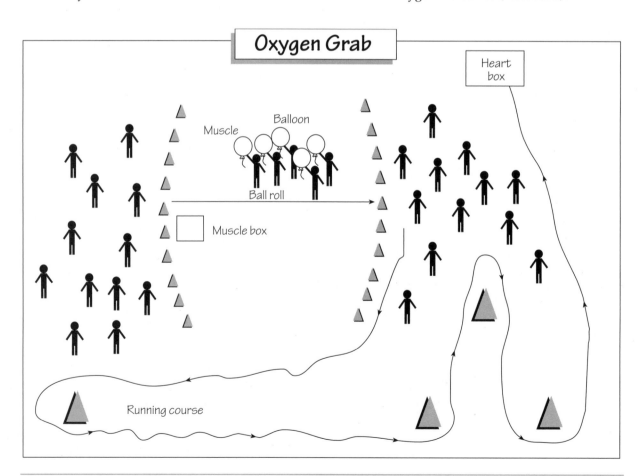

Fig. 1.4. Oxygen grab

- The blood cells roll a Nerf ball on the ground, across the muscle to the other blood cells.
- The muscle cells try to intercept the oxygen while keeping a balloon in the air. After intercepting the oxygen, it is placed in a box in the muscle.
- A blood cell student can retrieve a ball from the heart box when a muscle cell student intercepts a ball.
- The activity continues until the muscle cells have collected all Nerf balls, or periodically take balls from the muscle box to the heart box to keep the activity going. Rotate students into the muscle.

Cool-Down: 5 Minutes

Select stretching and cool-down activities.

Teaching Tips

Balls must be rolled. Establish a running course for blood cells returning to the heart to pick up an oxygen molecule. Often tennis clubs give away used balls.

Lesson 5

Feeling Fats

WEEK 1

Goals

- To introduce animal and plant fat
- To reinforce food categorization

Key Concepts

We all need some fat in the food we eat. Fat provides many healthy ingredients, such as vitamins, essential oils, and energy, and is used by the body to make tissues. Most of the fat we eat each day, such as meat, butter, whole milk, and cheese, comes from animals. Most plants have little, if any, fat. Fats derived from plants include oils such as corn, canola, and olive. A diet high in fat, both animal and plant, can make us gain weight, which will make the heart pump harder and can lead to heart disease. The problem with eating too much animal fat is that it can block the arteries and possibly result in heart attacks. It is important to eat a diet that is low in both animal and plant fats.

Materials

1. Paper towel tubing (six inches)
2. Modeling clay
3. Handout 1.1 Feeling Fats and matching overhead
4. Samples of food such as peanut butter, fruits, nuts, vegetables, breads, and cheese

5. Handout 1.2 Week 1, Family Activity: Hit the Mark (one per student)

Activity: Feeling Fats

- Before class, prepare a simulated blood vessel buildup by using a small piece of paper towel tubing (approximately six inches) and clay blocking the "artery."
- Brainstorm with the students about what foods, such as margarine, peanut butter, and meat, contain fat. As a group, classify several examples of common foods with obvious plant and animal sources. Which ones contain fat? Is the fat from animal or plant food?
- Show the students the "blocked blood vessel" and describe how eating too much animal fat can cause buildup. Also be sure to emphasize the need to reduce all fats, including plant fats.
- After assigning students to groups of two or three, instruct them, using handout 1.1, to test the samples of foods for fat using the "feel test." Next to the food, indicate whether they think the food came from an animal or a plant. Descriptive terms such as oily, creamy, or greasy can be used to identify the foods with fat. Indicate by a check which foods have fat. Do they see a pattern of food groups without fat (most animal foods have fat)?

- After the "feel test" has been completed, guide the students through the rest of the foods listed on the handout.
- When the list is completed, ask the students if they can guess whether their favorite foods contain fat (other than the ones listed).

Teaching Tips

Have samples of foods that contain fat to show the students, such as the layer of fat on top of old-fashioned peanut butter.

Answer key to handout 1.1: the foods without fat are banana, egg white, apple, carrots, potato, and oatmeal.

Handout 1.1   Feeling Fats

Which of the following foods do you think contain fat? Use the "feel test" for some of these foods to decide. If the food contains fat, it may feel creamy, oily, or greasy. If you think the food contains fat, put a check mark in the blank space provided.

Food	Contains Fat	
	Yes	No
Peanut butter	____	____
Tortilla	____	____
Banana	____	____
Processed meat	____	____
Egg yolk	____	____
Egg white	____	____
Chocolate	____	____
Apples	____	____
Avocado	____	____
Carrots	____	____
Potato	____	____
Oatmeal	____	____
Cheese	____	____

Handout 1.2   Week 1, Family Activity: Hit the Mark

Select any physical activity that you can do with a friend, family member, or neighbor. Your activity options can include walking, rope jumping, bicycling, swimming, soccer, basketball, dancing, and jogging. For every minute that you are active, you score a point. Use the fitness point chart to check off the minutes. Try to reach 100 points this week at home.

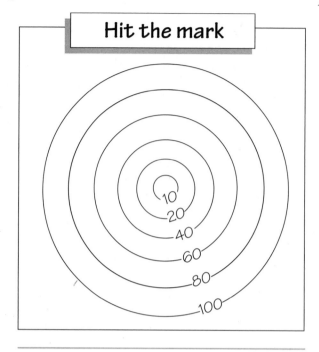

Fig. 1.5.   Hit the mark

Activity	Time	Points
_____	_____	_____
_____	_____	_____
_____	_____	_____
_____	_____	_____
_____	_____	_____
_____	_____	_____
_____	_____	_____
_____	_____	_____

Transfer the points to fig. 1.5. Use a different color for each circle as you complete the points.

Time: 100 minutes

Please return by _____.

Week 2: What's in a Workout?

The lessons introduce taking a pulse rate and students learn how to take resting, workout, and cool-down pulse rates.

WEEK 2

Lesson 6

The Basic Beat

Goals

- To help children learn to take their pulse rate
- To compare active and resting pulse rates

Key Concepts

An important part of fitness development is monitoring pulse rates. You can do this by finding pulse points where arteries are close to the surface. At these points, you can feel the heart pushing blood through the body. The pulse rate is the number of times your heart beats each minute. The rate changes with activity levels. When you're calm and relaxed your pulse is resting and is slower. When you are active, scared, or excited it is at a peak and the heart beats faster, increasing the pulse rate.

Materials

1. Jump ropes (one per student)
2. Two cups water
3. Cards or slips of paper
4. Poster board

Activity: The Basic Beat

To find the pulse, place your index and middle fingers (see fig. 2.1) on your wrist (radial artery) or neck (carotid artery). Do not use the thumb. The pulse in your thumb may be strong enough to interfere with your count. Hold your fingers in place until you feel the steady beat of your pulse. Most children can find their pulse after some activity. Play a tag game (see lesson 8) or have children jump rope for three or four minutes. This will increase the pulse rate and help children to locate a pulse. Explain that pulse rates increase when they are active. Complete some gentle stretching exercises for a few minutes and ask students to find their pulse again. The pulse should be slower by now.

Teaching Tips

Explain that a higher pulse rate represents an increase in the amount of blood being pumped by

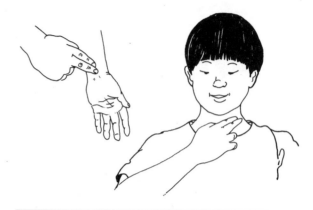

Fig. 2.1.   Taking a pulse

the heart. To illustrate use two cups, one with just a little water, the other full of water (as shown in fig. 2.2). Explain that during exercise, the amount of blood being pumped increases. Students can calculate their resting and active pulse rates by counting their pulse for 6 seconds and multiplying by 10. As a check ask them to count for 30 sec-

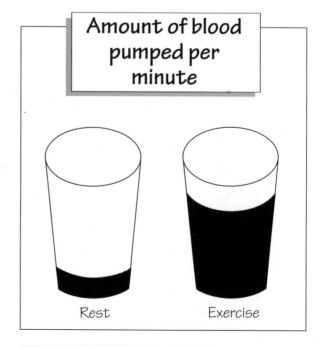

Amount of blood pumped per minute

Rest   Exercise

Fig. 2.2.   Blood pumped at rest and during exercise

onds and multiply by 2. Ask students to brainstorm a list of sports and physical activities. Encourage students to select activities that are vigorous and will provide 20 minutes of continuous activity. Discuss how some activities may be fun and enjoyable but not very active and, therefore, they do not make a good workout. Organize students into groups of four or five. Write the selected activities on cards or slips of paper. If students have not selected these activities, make sure to include jump rope, soccer, jogging, basketball,

swimming, bicycling, or rowing. One student from each group selects a workout topic. Each group will design a five-minute warm-up and a five-minute cool-down with their focus activity. Groups will then design a 5–20–5 poster that illustrates their complete workout, including warm-up, activity, and cool-down. Each group can share workouts with the class. Start collecting milk carton labels for lesson 17 (Moving With Moo). You can obtain cartons from creameries.

WEEK 2

Lesson 7

Hearty Hoops

Goals

- To develop cardiovascular endurance
- To practice body awareness exercises with a hoop

Key Concepts

A study Dr. Jeremy Morris did over 35 years ago in London, England, found that heart disease death rates were lower in bus conductors than in bus drivers (London buses have two decks, an upper and a lower). Increased physical activity of the conductors, who spent their days going up and down stairs, was considered the reason for their lower rates of heart disease. In contrast, bus drivers spent most of their days sitting.

Materials

1. Music with a strong beat
2. Hoops (one per student)

Warm-Up: 5 Minutes

Select stretching and warm-up activities.

Activity: Hearty Hoops

- Use the music after students have learned a few basic hoop activities.

- Every student has a hoop. Students jog or run around play area and on a signal, they find a hoop. On "one," find a hoop and complete one push-up. On "two," find a hoop and complete two sit-ups. On "three," find a hoop and complete three mountain climbers. Additional numbers can be added. Use this activity throughout the lesson while completing the following.
- Place hands in the hoop and your feet outside the hoop. Walk feet around the hoop in one direction, then in the other direction.
- Use the hoop as a jump rope and see how many consecutive jumps you can make.
- Jump with two feet out of your hoop and land outside on two feet. Jump back in and land on two feet. Repeat using one foot in turn.
- Hop all the way around the hoop in one direction, then hop around in the other direction. Use the left foot, then the right foot.
- Hold the hoop around the waist and see if you can spin the hoop around the waist.
- Hold the hoop in an upright position. Using your preferred hand, roll the hoop so it moves forward. Roll the hoop and move around area with the hoop. Roll into the open spaces. Roll the hoop forward, then run ahead of it and catch it (for outside use only).
- Roll the hoop forward, allowing it to fall to the ground. Jump into it and complete 10 jumping jacks.

- Hold the hoop upright and make it spin around like a spinning top. Spin the hoop, touch one line or wall, and come back to the hoop before it stops spinning.
- Take away one hoop. Scatter hoops in area and tell students to jog (or hop, gallop, skip, slide). When the music stops, each student finds a hoop. The student without a hoop can select an exercise (e.g., jumping jacks or cross-country skiers), and each student completes five repetitions of the exercise.

Cool-Down: 5 Minutes

Select stretching and cool-down activities.

Teaching Tips

Demonstrate each specific activity. Encourage students to bend at the knee to make a soft landing when jumping. Hoops can be noisy, so instruct students to place hoops on the floor when listening to instructions. Provide adequate space for activities.

Lesson 8

Target Tag

Goals

- To improve cardiovascular endurance
- To practice taking pulse rates

Key Concepts

To improve the efficiency of the heart, the heart muscle has to be overloaded. Just as the arm muscles increase in size with weight training, the heart muscle has to be exercised to increase in size, strength, and efficiency. Therefore, the heart has to pump faster for a certain time. Improvement in heart efficiency is best achieved when working between 50 and 85 percent of capacity. The pulse rate is raised to a target range through exercise.

Materials

1. Nerf balls for taggers (five)
2. Cones (to mark out play areas)

Warm-Up: 5 Minutes

Select stretching and warm-up activities.

Activity: Target Tag

Complete the following tag games and take a break every few minutes for children to find their pulse rates. Review procedures from lesson 6 for taking pulse rates.

1. Ten-second tag
   - Make an area 30 × 30 yards or larger (depending on number of students).
   - Divide class in half with one group scattered in the area and the second group lined up along one line.
   - On signal, the first two students from the line run inside and have 10 seconds to tag a student.
   - If successful, they trade places with students tagged; if not, they get back in line.
2. Hug tag
   - Players are inside a court area marked by cones.
   - Two players stand outside court with Nerf balls for tagging.
   - On signal, the teacher calls out a number from 1 to 5. On 3, for example, players must get in groups of three (holding

hands, linking elbows, hugging) to be safe from taggers.

- If a player is tagged, he or she is immediately the new tagger and takes the Nerf ball.
- Every minute you can call a new number.

3. Blob tag

- Players are scattered inside a court area.
- Two players, holding hands, are the beginning blob. There can be two sets of blobs—a boy team and girl team works well.
- The blobs run around tagging other players with outside hands. As players are tagged, they become part of the blob.

4. Elbow tag

- Players are in twos with elbows locked together.
- Outside hands are placed on hips.
- One player is a tagger who chases pairs and tries to hook onto an outside elbow.
- The outside player on the other side becomes the new tagger.

Use the following chart to help children identify a target heart rate. Based on a resting heart rate, help children identify their target rate. The maximum heart rate is approximately 220 beats per minute minus a person's age. The target rate represents approximately 60 to 75 percent of the maximum rate.

Resting heart rate	Target heart rate
Below 60	150
60–64	151
65–69	153
70–74	155
75–79	157
80–84	159
85–89	161
90+	163

Cool-Down: 5 Minutes

Select stretching and cool-down activities.

Teaching Tips

Emphasize safety in tagging to avoid pushing and shoving.

WEEK 2

Lesson 9

Moving to the Beat

Goals

- To practice taking and computing pulse rates
- To improve cardiovascular endurance
- To teach basic locomotor movements of skipping, hopping, galloping, sliding, and leaping

Key Concepts

Exercise makes your pulse rate go up rapidly. Most of the change takes place during the first two minutes. After that the pulse rate goes up more slowly and levels off. When you stop exercising it drops back down. After easy exercise, the pulse rate slows quickly. If the exercise is long and hard, it will take 5 to 10 minutes to go down.

Materials

1. Four cones
2. Tennis balls or bean bags (optional)

Warm-Up: 5 Minutes

Select stretching and warm-up activities. Have students take pulse rates before warm-up.

Activity: Moving to the Beat

- Mark out a square area the size of a basketball court or larger with four cones. There needs to be enough space for students to run and jump.

- In the middle of the lesson stop and have children take their pulse rate. It should be close to their target rate as identified in lesson 8.
- Start with students walking in all directions.
- Tell students to run, first slowly, then gradually increase speed. They can experiment with varying the speed of the run.
- Emphasize changing pace and direction.
- Students can then run and jump and land, using a one-foot takeoff.
- Continue the lesson with these movements—skipping, hopping (using both feet), galloping, sliding (side to side movement), leaping.
- Change commands to vary patterns and rates of movements, such as fast and slow, forward and backward, changing the lead leg, moving in circular, square, and rectangular patterns on the floor.
- Ask children to develop their own sequence of movements, such as running and leaping, skipping slowly, galloping fast, and hopping on the left foot and backward. Different types of jumps (high, long, with a shape, rotate, one-foot takeoff, two-foot takeoff) can be introduced.
- Equipment, such as tennis balls and bean bags, may be introduced. For example, children can complete all movements while throwing and catching a tennis ball or bean bag. Bean bags or balls—throw and catch with one hand; throw and catch with two hands; jog, throw, and catch; jog, throw, make and shape, and catch; jog, throw, jump, and catch with one hand or two hands.

Cool-Down: 5 Minutes

Select stretching and cool-down activities.

Teaching Tips

Emphasize creative movement, not merely running around in a circle. Encourage using arms in opposition to the legs in all movements. Introduce animal walks to provide more variety.

WEEK 2

Lesson 10

Cookie Quest

Goals

- To recognize the fat source in cookies
- To prepare low-fat cookies

Key Concepts

Most children enjoy making and eating cookies. Unfortunately, cookies are often laden with fat. Drop cookies rely on solid fats for texture and flavor. If the fat is left out, cookies become tough and tasteless; fat provides color to cookies. You can reduce the amount of fat without losing flavor by replacing part of the fat with applesauce, nonfat yogurt, or pureed prunes. You can also use egg whites for texture because they do not contain fat as do egg yolks.

Materials

1. A copy of a traditional oatmeal cookie recipe (per group)
2. Low-fat oatmeal cookie recipe (per group)
3. Ingredients and equipment for baking oatmeal cookies
4. Handout 2.1 Week 2, Family Activity: The Beat Goes Home (one per student)

Activity: Cookie Quest

- Explain to students the objectives of today's lesson. Ask them if they know what fat provides to food (texture and flavor).
- Place the students in groups and give each student a traditional oatmeal cookie recipe.

Ask them to circle the ingredients that contain fat (shortening, oil, eggs).

- Next, provide them with the low-fat oatmeal cookie recipe. How does it differ from the traditional cookie recipe?
- Instruct the students to make a batch of low-fat cookies and discuss the results.

Low-Fat Oatmeal Cookies

1 cup packed brown sugar
3/4 cup unsweetened applesauce
1 egg white, lightly beaten
2 T. vegetable oil
1 T. vanilla extract
1 cup raisins
2 cup rolled oats
1 cup sifted cake flour
1/2 cup whole wheat flour
1/2 T. baking soda
1 tsp. ground cinnamon
1/2 tsp. salt
Bake at 350° F for 8 to 10 minutes.

Handout 2.1   Week 2, Family Activity: The Beat Goes Home

Students, teach your family members how to take their pulse rates. In this activity, each family member will take their pulse rate while reading or sitting down. Family members retake their pulse rate during light activity, such as walking. Students record the pulse of each family member.

Family member's name

Pulse				
Resting	_____	_____	_____	_____
Activity ( )	_____	_____	_____	_____
Activity ( )	_____	_____	_____	_____
Activity ( )	_____	_____	_____	_____

Time: 25 minutes

Please return by _____.

Week 3: Fitness Components

Physical fitness testing precedes activities that help students distinguish different fitness components. The lesson on nutrition emphasizes drinking water to replenish body fluids.

WEEK 3

Lesson 11

Fit Kids

Goal

- To assess physical fitness levels of students in muscular strength and endurance, flexibility, and cardiovascular endurance

Key Concepts

Cardiovascular endurance, low-back and posterior thigh flexibility, abdominal endurance, and upper body muscular strength and endurance are basic components of physical fitness. In this lesson, test items measure each fitness component.

Materials

1. Stopwatch
2. Sit-and-reach box or yardstick or measuring tape, and masking tape
3. Mats
4. Handout 3.1 Fit Kids Score Sheet

Warm-Up: 5 Minutes

Select stretching and warm-up activities.

Activity: Fit Kids

Test children on the following items:

1. *Mile run (cardiovascular endurance test)*
   The score is the time in minutes and seconds to run the mile. Instruct students to run or walk at the fastest pace possible. This test needs to be practiced several times before testing to develop confidence and a sense of pacing. Divide into pairs and complete in two separate groups with partners serving as recorders of time.

2. *Sit and reach (lower-back and thigh flexibility test)*
   Use a sit-and-reach box (see figure 3.1) or a yardstick or measuring tape. If using a yardstick or measuring tape, put a piece of masking tape on the floor. Students sit perpendicular to it with legs extended, knees straight, heels five to seven inches apart and just

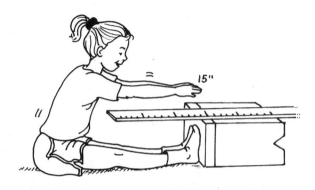

Fig. 3.1.   Sit and reach

touching the inside edge of the tape. Place a yardstick or measuring tape between legs with the 15-inch mark on the inside edge of the masking tape. A partner holds the student's knees straight. Student places both hands on top of each other with tips of fingers matching, then reaches forward with both hands as far as possible, touches the stick, and holds for a second. Record the score to the nearest half inch.

3. *Sit-ups (abdominal muscular endurance test)*
   Student lies on back with knees flexed and feet flat on floor. Heels are between 12 and 18 inches from buttocks. The arms are crossed on the chest with the hands on opposite shoulders. A partner holds the feet to keep them in contact with the ground. The student curls to the sitting position. The student must maintain arm contact with chest. The chin remains tucked on the chest. The sit-up is completed when the elbows touch the thighs. The student returns to the down position until the midback makes contact with the surface of the mat (to complete the movement). The score is the number of correctly completed sit-ups in one minute.

4. *Push-ups (upper body muscular strength and endurance test)*
   Student lies on stomach with chest touching the floor. The hands are directly under the shoulders, fingers pointing forward. The student raises body by fully extending the arms and then lowers to starting position. Raise

and lower the body in a straight line, not allowing the back to sway. The score is the number of correctly completed push-ups in 30 seconds.

Cool-Down: 5 Minutes

Select stretching and cool-down activities.

Teaching Tips

Students can work in pairs and take turns testing each other and recording scores. Students will obviously compare scores and there is a need to emphasize that scores are a baseline measure and individual improvement is the goal. This lesson is more than one 30-minute period. You may need to spread it out over a few days. Students need to practice running in previous lessons before completing the mile run. You can repeat the tests at the end of the year or periodically during the year. Students practice measurement skills by marking out a 70 × 40 yd. rectangle for the mile run. Eight laps equals one mile. Have students compute total class laps into miles.

Handout 3.1   Fit Kids Score Sheet

Name	Mile run		Sit and reach		Sit-ups		Push-ups	
	Test 1	Test 2	Test 1	Test 2	Test 1	Test 2	Test 1	Test 2
1. _____	_____	_____	_____	_____	_____	_____	_____	_____
2. _____	_____	_____	_____	_____	_____	_____	_____	_____
3. _____	_____	_____	_____	_____	_____	_____	_____	_____
4. _____	_____	_____	_____	_____	_____	_____	_____	_____
5. _____	_____	_____	_____	_____	_____	_____	_____	_____
6. _____	_____	_____	_____	_____	_____	_____	_____	_____
7. _____	_____	_____	_____	_____	_____	_____	_____	_____
8. _____	_____	_____	_____	_____	_____	_____	_____	_____
9. _____	_____	_____	_____	_____	_____	_____	_____	_____
10. _____	_____	_____	_____	_____	_____	_____	_____	_____
11. _____	_____	_____	_____	_____	_____	_____	_____	_____
12. _____	_____	_____	_____	_____	_____	_____	_____	_____
13. _____	_____	_____	_____	_____	_____	_____	_____	_____
14. _____	_____	_____	_____	_____	_____	_____	_____	_____
15. _____	_____	_____	_____	_____	_____	_____	_____	_____
16. _____	_____	_____	_____	_____	_____	_____	_____	_____
17. _____	_____	_____	_____	_____	_____	_____	_____	_____
18. _____	_____	_____	_____	_____	_____	_____	_____	_____
19. _____	_____	_____	_____	_____	_____	_____	_____	_____
20. _____	_____	_____	_____	_____	_____	_____	_____	_____
21. _____	_____	_____	_____	_____	_____	_____	_____	_____
22. _____	_____	_____	_____	_____	_____	_____	_____	_____
23. _____	_____	_____	_____	_____	_____	_____	_____	_____
24. _____	_____	_____	_____	_____	_____	_____	_____	_____
25. _____	_____	_____	_____	_____	_____	_____	_____	_____
26. _____	_____	_____	_____	_____	_____	_____	_____	_____
27. _____	_____	_____	_____	_____	_____	_____	_____	_____
28. _____	_____	_____	_____	_____	_____	_____	_____	_____
29. _____	_____	_____	_____	_____	_____	_____	_____	_____
30. _____	_____	_____	_____	_____	_____	_____	_____	_____

WEEK 3

Lesson 12

Fitness Quest

Goal

- To categorize exercise activities into muscular strength and endurance, flexibility, and endurance fitness components

Key Concepts

Cardiovascular fitness that improves the efficiency of the heart and lungs is often considered the most important fitness component. However, muscular strength and endurance and flexibility are important fitness components to develop in children. Most importantly, children need to understand how they can improve these components. Although we lose these characteristics more slowly as we age than we lose cardiovascular endurance, low levels of strength and flexibility ultimately prevent carrying out daily activities.

Materials

1. Handout 3.2 Fitness Quest sheet
2. Jump ropes
3. Cones
4. Nerf ball for tag game
5. Basketballs (eight)

Warm-Up: 5 Minutes

Select stretching and warm-up activities.

Activity: Fitness Quest

- Children complete the list of activities included on the Fitness Quest sheet.
- Children name the fitness component measured by each activity.

- Teach children to recognize the different physical effort required by each activity. Use the following characteristics of each type of exercise as your students evaluate each activity.

Characteristics of cardiovascular activities

- Continuous, not stop and start
- Uses large muscles of body
- Increases breathing
- Rhythmic
- Can do for 10 to 15 minutes or longer
- Examples: jogging, bicycling

Characteristics of flexibility exercises

- Slow, deliberate, and controlled movements
- Stretches specific joints in the body
- Move body part until tension is felt in the muscle
- Hold for 5 to 15 seconds
- Examples: any stretching activity in Routines 1, 2, 3 (see chapter 10)

Characteristics of muscular strength and endurance exercises

- Very physically demanding
- Can only do for a short time (one minute)
- Uses certain muscle groups, not whole body
- Examples: sit-ups, crunches, pull-ups, mountain climbers, push-ups

Cool-Down: 5 Minutes

Select stretching and cool-down activities.

Teaching Tips

The teacher can organize the lesson in a station format or lead the class through each activity in turn.

Handout 3.2   Fitness Quest

Activity	Fitness component
1. Jogging for three minutes around cones	CE
2. Climbing a rope (if available)	MSE
3. Jumping rope for three minutes	CE
4. Sitting stretch (see Stretching Routine 3, in chapter 10)	F
5. Tag game (two minutes of freeze tag)	CE
6. Crab legs (10)*	MSE
7. Crunches (10)*	MSE
8. Low-back stretch (see Stretching Routine 2, in chapter 10)	F
9. Two versus two basketball for three minutes (or similar activity)	CE

*In chapter 13

Key: Muscular strength and endurance   MSE

Flexibility   F

Cardiovascular Endurance   CE

Lesson 13

25 Ways to Fitness

Goals

- To improve cardiovascular fitness
- To improve muscular strength and endurance

Key Concepts

Daily weight-bearing activities are critical for enhancing bone development that affects skeletal health. The foundation of bone health begins early in life and exercise increases bone mass up to, and through, adolescence.

Materials

1. Handout 3.3 Fitness Grid
2. Jump ropes (one per student)
3. A deck of cards using only ace through five of each suit

Warm-Up: 5 minutes

Select stretching and warm-up activities.

Activity: 25 Ways to Fitness

- Use the grid of 25 activities in handout 3.3. Show the grid to the class and make sure everyone understands each activity.

- Divide class into five squads with a designated line-up format. Each squad spreads out to ensure a gap of two or three yards between each student.
- Deal two cards to each squad in turn.
- The first card indicates the horizontal number on the grid, the second card indicates the vertical number.
- The squad leader finds the correct activity, and tells the squad the activity to perform.
- When students are finished, they stand in line in their squads. After every deal the squad leader moves to the back of the line and a new squad leader is assigned.

Cool-Down: 5 Minutes

Select stretching and cool-down activities.

Teaching Tips

Often airlines give away packs of cards. Oversize playing cards are an option and are available at novelty shops. Alternatively, students can design their own cards. Squads cannot enter an area where children are doing an exercise. See chapter 13 for exercise descriptions.

Handout 3.3   Fitness Grid

	1	2	3	4	5
1	20 sit-ups	20 jump ropes	Touch 4 lines (one group at a time)	10 jumping jacks	Take a rest
2	Hop on left foot 20 times	10 jack-in-the-boxes	30 jump ropes (any style)	Run in place for 1 minute	5 mountain climbers
3	Jog in place for 25 seconds	10 reverse push-ups	40 jump ropes (any style)	5 squat thrusts	15 stride jumps
4	5 reverse push-ups	5 crunches	10 cross-country skiers	5 push-ups	50 jump ropes (single bounce)
5	Take a rest	10 side leg raises	25 clappers	10 chest raises	30 jump ropes (double bounce)

Lesson 14

02 (Oh-Two)

Goals

- To improve cardiovascular fitness
- To reinforce the role oxygen plays in healthy body systems

Key Concepts

Intense, continuous, and vigorous activity increases heart rate and blood flow. The heart and all muscles in the body need a supply of oxygen to function efficiently. Oxygen is transported in the blood to the muscles. Explain to children that a shortness of breath after or during exercise is because the lungs have to get more oxygen to the muscles of the body for the muscles to keep working.

Materials

1. Hoops (five or six)
2. Bean bags or balls (25–30)

Warm-Up: 5 minutes

Select stretching and warm-up activities.

Activity: 02 (Oh-Two)

- Divide the students into groups of four or five.
- Arrange hoops equal distances from each other.

- Place four or five bean bags on the ground, in the hoops.
- Each group has a home base (one of the hula hoops).
- On the signal to start the game, players try to steal an oxygen molecule (bean bag) from another team, and bring it back to their home base.
- Each student is allowed to carry only one oxygen molecule at a time. There is no guarding of home base. Students may take a molecule from the hoop of any or all of the teams.
- Oxygen molecules may not be passed or thrown.
- After three minutes, give the command "Freeze", and each team counts the number of captured oxygen molecules.
- Emphasize that all strong hearts need a good supply of oxygen for efficiency.

Cool-Down: 5 Minutes

Select stretching and cool-down activities.

Teaching Tips

Have the students perform different aerobic activities besides running, such as hopping, skipping, and race-walking. Do not allow students to guard their own hoop or throw bean bags around room. Change makeup of groups if necessary.

Lesson 15

Body of Water

Goals

- To reinforce the human body's need for water
- To introduce body composition as it relates to water

Key Concepts

The human body is composed primarily of water. In fact, water represents 50 to 75 percent of a person's body weight. The percentage of water fluctuates depending on muscle mass (the more muscle, the higher the amount of body water). Typically children have a smaller percentage of water because they have less muscle mass and more body fat than adults. Water regulates body temperature. The body's need for water is second only to its need for oxygen. One can live for an extended period without food, but not without water.

The primary ways the body loses water are through urination and perspiration. The primary methods for replenishing needed water are through eating and drinking. You can meet daily water requirements by drinking six to eight cups of water per day.

Materials

1. One pitcher and 12 eight-ounce paper cups (per group)
2. Fig. 3.2 (one per student)
3. Fig. 3.3
4. Handout 3.4 Week 3, Family Activity: Century March (one per student)

Activity: Body of Water

- Describe to the students the objective of the lesson. Include expectations and content of the lesson.
- Explain the lesson concepts. Complete fig. 3.2 using overhead transparency. Figure 3.3 shows how fig. 3.2 should be completed.
- Organize students into groups of three or four. Designate the following responsibilities: materials manager, water person, cleanup, and reporter. Give each group a pitcher of water and several eight-ounce paper cups. Have students discuss daily amount of water needed and indicate their response by filling in the appropriate number of cups with water.
- Ask each group to share their results and thinking.
- Give feedback at the end of sharing and have each group adjust their responses.
- Instruct each student to drink one eight-ounce cup and discuss their feelings: Are they full? When might you drink more than

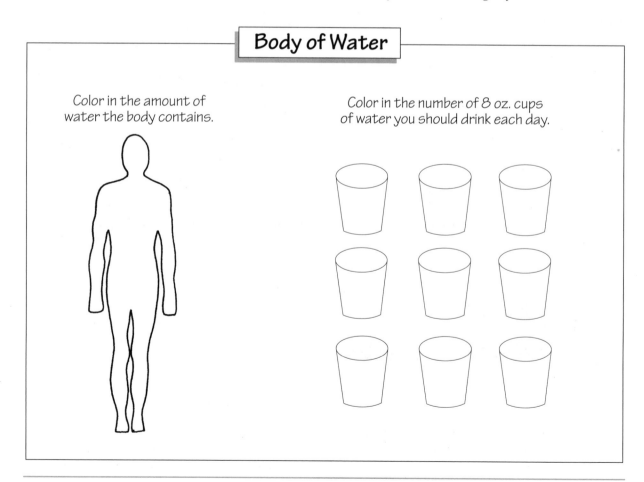

Fig. 3.2. Water in the body

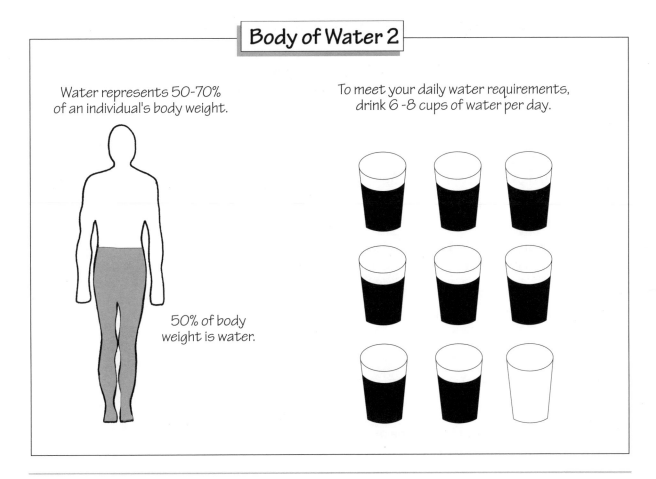

Body of Water 2

Water represents 50-70% of an individual's body weight.

To meet your daily water requirements, drink 6-8 cups of water per day.

50% of body weight is water.

Fig. 3.3. Water in the body—completed outline

one cup of water? Do you think you are drinking more or less than eight ounces at the drinking fountain?

Teaching Tips

Provide trays for easy handout and cleanup of materials. If the teacher is concerned about spills, have the students predict using cups without water. Have students keep a "water log" for 24 hours. Create a classroom bar graph with the results.

Handout 3.4   Week 3, Family Activity: Century March

Complete the following activities to gain 100 points in the next two weeks. Each activity is worth 10 points. Write in the date that you completed the activities. You can repeat activities.

Activity	Points	Date
1. Miss one of your favorite TV shows and go outside to play for 15 minutes.	_____	_____
2. Help a parent with an outside chore.	_____	_____
3. Help sweep or clean a part of the house for 5 to 10 minutes.	_____	_____
4. Find someone (friend or brother or sister) to play a ball game.	_____	_____
5. Do 15 sit-ups and push-ups.	_____	_____
6. Take the stairs instead of elevator or escalator.	_____	_____
7. Take a bike ride.	_____	_____
8. Walk to store instead of driving.	_____	_____
9. Plan a healthy picnic or meal.	_____	_____
10. Complete 10 minutes of jump rope or jog twice around the block or 10 times around yard.	_____	_____

Start date _____

End date _____

Time: 10 to 15 minutes per activity

Please return by _____.

CHAPTER

4

Week 4: Risk Factors

The lessons examine the role of exercise in preventing or reducing cardiovascular disease. The nutrition lesson introduces salt in the diet and strategies to reduce salt in food.

WEEK 4

Lesson 16
Staying Active

Goal

- To help students develop plans for an active lifestyle

Key Concepts

Inactivity is one of the major risk factors for heart disease. Therefore, teaching students how to stay active helps to reduce the likelihood of heart disease later in life. According to Steven N. Blair of the Cooper Institute for Aerobics Research, inactive lifestyles pose a major health risk. Blair notes, "It's alarming that 40 to 50 million American adults are sedentary, and this places them at a substantially increased risk for heart attacks, some cancers, and chronic diseases."

Materials

Handout 4.1 My Plan for Staying Active (one per student)

Activity: Staying Active

Adults sometimes suffer from heart disease and are at risk for a heart attack. Although children generally do not have heart attacks, they can help protect themselves by staying active and reducing the risk of a heart attack later in life. Describe the signs of heart attack to children: discomfort or pain in chest area; pain spreading to shoulders, neck, and arms; lightheadedness, fainting, sweating, or shortness of breath.

Explain that exercise can reduce the chances of having a heart attack. Exercise, especially the type that is continuous and uses large muscle groups in the body helps to delay heart disease. Therefore, staying active is good for your health. Inactive people have almost twice the risk of developing heart disease as active people.

There are many ways to stay active. One way is to play sports. Another alternative is to complete chores, such as raking leaves in the fall. Yet another strategy is to play games or do exercise at home. Students can complete My Plan for Staying Active. Younger children can color pictures. Older children can draw and write in their plans. Students can present a plan to the class after working in pairs and reporting to each other on their responses to the questions.

Teaching Tips

Help children recognize some of the barriers to exercise, such as time, equipment, and space. Help children develop strategies to overcome some of the barriers. You could revisit this lesson later in the year with responses that demonstrate growth. Staying Active Plans can be kept in a portfolio.

Handout 4.1   My Plan for Staying Active

Sports I would like to learn:

Active things I can do instead of watching TV:

Ways I can help around the home and increase my physical activity:

Things to do in summertime, weekends, or holidays that are active:

WEEK 4

Lesson 17

Moving With Moo

Goals

- To improve cardiovascular endurance
- To demonstrate varying fat levels in different types of milk

Key Concepts

A major source of saturated fat in the typical American diet is dairy products. Whole milk is a high-fat food. Different types of milk contain varying amounts of fat. Learning to read labels teaches students to recognize the fat levels in the various types of milk.

Materials

1. Empty milk carton labels of whole, 2 percent, 1 percent, and skim milk (four each)
2. Four large paper bags
3. Cones to mark out playing areas

Warm-Up: 5 Minutes

Select stretching and warm-up activities.

Activity: Moving With Moo

- In class ahead of time, explain the fat content of different types of milk.
- Set up four rectangles with cones as shown in fig. 4.1.
- The largest rectangle is 50 × 30 yards.
- Inside this rectangle is a smaller rectangle 40 × 25 yards.
- Mark out other rectangles, 35 × 15 and 30 × 10 yards, inside the bigger rectangles.

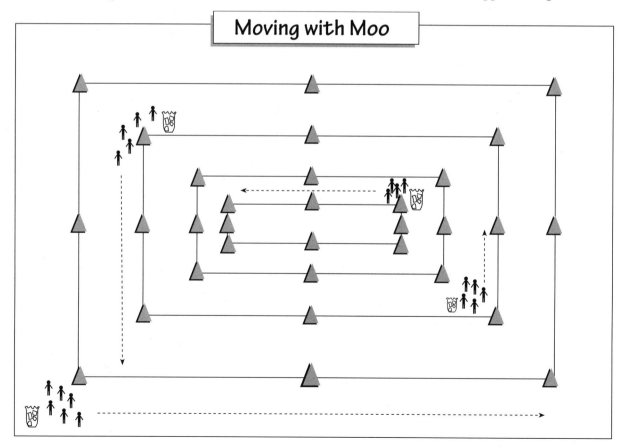

Fig. 4.1.   Moving with Moo

- Use empty milk carton labels (four each of whole, 2 percent, 1 percent, and skim) and write on the label with a black pen the number of grams of fat in an eight-ounce glass of milk [whole (eight), 2 percent (five), 1 percent (three), skim (zero)].
- Write the name of an exercise on the back of each label. Place one of each in a paper bag.
- Divide the class into four equal groups, one at a corner of each square.
- Without looking, one player from each team picks out a milk carton label.
- The number of grams of fat is the number of segments (one side of the square) that students run in each group. For example, if the player picks a whole milk carton label, the team will run eight segments.
- The team then completes repetitions of the designated exercise (on the back of the label) before picking the next label. If the team selected whole milk, they complete eight repetitions. If they selected 2 percent milk, they complete five repetitions.

- Rotate children around different sized squares after four minutes.

Cool-Down: 5 Minutes

Select stretching and cool-down activities.

Teaching Tips

You can copy labels to avoid collecting many labels. Use exercises described in chapter 13. This is a demanding activity, so provide a break and discuss the number of grams of fat in different types of milk. Use cards with the type of milk and number of grams of fat written on them if carton labels are unavailable. Students can complete a survey by rating the milk in their refrigerators for fat. Students can then graph the results. Also, children can calculate container size to determine total amounts of fat in each container. They can compute average consumption for class and family members.

WEEK 4

Lesson 18

Jump Start

Goals

- To improve jump rope skills
- To improve cardiovascular endurance

Key Concepts

The American Heart Association and the American Alliance for Health, Physical Education, Recreation and Dance sponsor Jump Rope for Heart. Jumping rope is an activity that rapidly increases heart rate and allows students to reach target heart rate levels. It is easy to do and many students enjoy the activity.

Materials

1. Jump ropes (one for each student)
2. Music and tape player

Warm-Up: 5 Minutes

Select stretching and warm-up activities.

Activity: Jump Start

- Use an audiotape that has repeated intervals of 30 seconds of music followed by 45 seconds of silence.
- When the music plays, students jump rope.
- At more advanced fitness levels when silence occurs, children perform exercises (use exercises in chapter 13, such as jumping jacks).
- Challenge children to try different jump rope routines such as single bounce, skier (side to side) and bell (forward and back).
- Students can take their pulse rates at varying times throughout the workout.

Cool-Down: 5 Minutes

Select stretching and cool-down activities.

Teaching Tips

To prevent fatigue, silence periods can serve as a rest period. Consecutive exercises should not use the same body parts (sit-ups and crunches work the abdominal muscle area and students should not complete one after another). Introduce students to jump rope rhymes to provide an active way for them to develop oral language skills. This is also an excellent way to improve memory skills.

Lesson 19

Save Your Heart

WEEK 4

Goals

- To develop upper body strength
- To improve cardiovascular fitness
- To develop throwing skills

Key Concepts

Two primary factors that contribute to heart disease are physical inactivity and a diet high in saturated fat and cholesterol. Both factors are controllable and can be adjusted through lifestyle changes.

Materials

1. Forty foam balls (or as many as you have)
2. Six cones
3. Two boxes

Warm-Up: 5 Minutes

Select stretching and warm-up activities.

Activity: Save Your Heart

- Mark out a playing area 30 × 30 yards (see fig. 4.2).
- Divide the class into two teams with a centerline between each team.
- Give each team 20 foam balls. Mark each ball with the name of a food or activity.
- The objective of the game is for each team to keep the foam balls that are likely to reduce the risk of a heart attack and get rid of the balls that may cause a heart attack.
- If a ball has the name of a food or activity that may put a person at risk, the player throws that ball into the opposing team's playing area.
- Designate a box in a safe area behind the playing area of the opposing teams for each

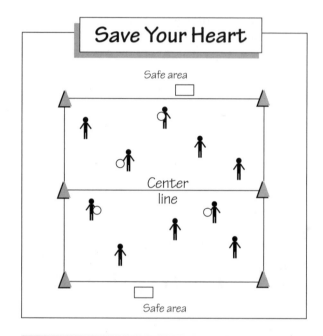

Fig. 4.2.   Save your heart

team to collect balls that have names of food or activities that prevent heart attacks.
- The player runs through the opposing team and drops the ball into the box.
- If tagged going through, the player releases the ball and returns to own side.
- If players make it through to the box, they cannot be tagged returning to their own team.
- Play for four minutes, stop and see who has the most balls in the box. Then restart the activity.

Cool-Down: 5 Minutes

Select stretching and cool-down activities.

Teaching Tips

Use a felt-tip pen or marker to write names of foods or activities on masking tape to place on the balls. The following would be "keeper" balls: vegetables, fruits, jogging, bicycling, low-fat milk, rice, potatoes, fish, sit-ups, and pasta. The following would be examples of throw-away balls: watching TV, hot dogs, french fries, fried foods, and butter.

WEEK 4

Lesson 20

Salt Solution

Goals

- To understand the need for salt in the human body
- To reinforce the need for drinking water

Key Concepts

Some salt is necessary for the human body, but excessive amounts can be damaging. One major function of salt is to keep body water in balance. Excessive amounts of salt may result in greater amounts of body water. Salt is used in processed foods as a flavor enhancer and preservative. Many processed foods contain levels of salt that exceed minimum daily requirements.

Materials

1. One bag unsalted popcorn marked A (one per student group)
2. One bag salted popcorn marked B (one per student group)
3. One bag unsalted popcorn marked C (one per student group)
4. One eight-ounce cup of water per student
5. Handout 4.2 Week 4, Family Activity: Sports Cards

6. Six-by-nine-inch index cards (two per student)

Activity: Salt Solution

- Review the information from lesson 15 concerning the minimum daily requirement of water.
- If students have kept a water log, have them share their results and create a classroom bar graph.
- Organize students into groups of three or four. Hand out bags A, B, and C to each group. Have students sample A. Take a drink of water to clear the palate. Continue with samples B and C.
- Discuss their personal findings. What do they think is the difference between the samples? Do any of the samples increase drinking? Which sample tasted the best?
- Share group discussion with class. Reinforce the concept that the body requires greater water intake after eating salty foods because of the greater concentration of salt in the blood.

Handout 4.2   Week 4, Family Activity: Sports Cards

Illustrate two sports activities on six-by-nine index cards. Use magazine pictures or your own drawings to illustrate one side of the card. Leave the other side blank. Each card should focus on only one activity or sport. Do not combine sports on a card or label the cards. These cards will be used in activities at school. Select activities that your family enjoys.

Time: 15 minutes

Please return by _____.

CHAPTER 5

Week 5: Aerobic Fitness

The lessons explain the concept of aerobic exercise and its distinctive characteristics. The nutrition information further develops the role of salt.

WEEK 5

Lesson 21

Aerobic Pacing

Goals

- To identify activities that are physically demanding and require oxygen to perform
- To compare and contrast aerobic and nonaerobic activities

Key Concepts

Aerobic exercise requires the heart and lungs to work hard and improves the efficiency of the cardiovascular system. Aerobic exercise requires continuous movement, lasts longer than 90 seconds, and increases the supply of oxygen to the muscles. Not all activities are aerobic. Those that can be continuous and use the large muscles of the body such as bicycling, swimming, and running are aerobic.

Materials

1. Four cones
2. Stopwatch

Warm-Up: 5 Minutes

Select stretching and warm-up activities.

Activity: Aerobic Pacing

Aerobic exercise requires the heart and lungs to work harder than normal. Therefore, activities that can be done for an extended time such as swimming, running, and bicycling are known as

aerobic. Play a short game of kickball (one inning) with your class. Then set up a course for running (200 yards). Use four cones to mark out running course. Establish a time period for your class to run based on their grade level. The objective is for students to keep running for the entire time. We suggest the following intervals: five minutes for third grade, six minutes for fourth grade. Emphasize the goal of this activity is running or moving at a pace that is comfortable. If students ran so hard they had to stop and catch their breath, it was not aerobic exercise.

Ask students to compare activities (kickball and running).

Are the two activities similar in effort?

Which activity required your heart and lungs to work harder?

How much time in kickball did you spend moving?

Students can write a short paragraph about the difference between aerobic and nonaerobic activities.

Cool-Down: 5 Minutes

Select stretching and cool-down activities.

Teaching Tips

Start runners at different points on the course so it does not appear to be a race. Starting runners at a common point can show who are the slowest and fastest runners. Those who fall behind may not give their best efforts.

WEEK 5

Lesson 22

Target Fitness I

Goals

- To predict performance on fitness activities
- To measure current performance levels

Key Concepts

Learning to predict and estimate performance provides a foundation for an individualized approach to exercise. Children predict their scores and then set a realistic new goal based on actual performance. In most cases changes in fitness levels are limited over a short time. However, staying with exercise over a longer time (6–10 weeks) can produce substantial improvements.

Materials

1. Mats
2. Stopwatch
3. Handout 5.1 Target Fitness Sheet (one per student)

Warm-Up: 5 Minutes

Select stretching and warm-up activities.

Activity: Target Fitness I

- Use the Target Fitness Sheet and help students estimate the number of exercises they can perform in one-minute periods.

- Students then complete the exercises.
- Use the sheet to help them set realistic new goals.
- This lesson is repeated in lesson 32.
- Children should be familiar with each exercise and have previously practiced the exercise.

Cool-Down: 5 Minutes

Select stretching and cool-down activities.

Teaching Tips

Set up stations for activities. Children may work individually or in pairs. As a basis for determining their performance levels, provide a brief practice period for all children to try the exercises. Make sure they use correct technique. Do not allow children to count exercises that are performed incorrectly. Although children are unlikely to see great changes in two weeks, a little improvement is realistic.

Handout 5.1   Target Fitness Sheet

Name_____   Dates_____

Exercise	Number predicted	Number performed	Revised goal	Second performance
Push-ups or modified push-ups	_____	_____	_____	_____
Side leg raises	_____	_____	_____	_____
Mountain climbers	_____	_____	_____	_____
Sit-ups	_____	_____	_____	_____
Jumping jacks	_____	_____	_____	_____
Reverse push-ups	_____	_____	_____	_____

You can add or substitute other exercises.

Lesson 23

Fortune Fitness

Goals

- To improve muscular strength and endurance
- To improve cardiovascular endurance

Key Concepts

Building small, incremental physical activities into a daily routine can have significant benefits in both weight loss and weight maintenance programs and fitness programs. The total accumulation of energy expenditure is what is important. Do not worry about achieving a specific dose of exercise, but focus on increasing activity levels. Modest increases in activity will produce changes in fitness.

Materials

Pieces of paper with tasks or activities written on them

Warm-Up: 5 Minutes

Select stretching and warm-up activities.

Activity: Fortune Fitness

- Before class write down a variety of tasks on pieces of paper.
- Divide class into five teams.
- Each team takes a turn in selecting a piece of paper.

- All the teams complete the task and then line up.
- Another team selects a new fortune piece.
- You can use the following tasks: crab walk the across the gym, then give four players a crab walk greeting (touching the bottom of your shoe to the bottom of another player's); run three laps clockwise around the play area; complete eight sit-ups in each corner; imitate the swim strokes (front crawl, backstroke, breaststroke) while jogging three circuits in a clockwise route.
- Include the following as examples of how children can increase the physical activity in their lives: jogging in place, stair stepping, line jumps, bicycling (lying on back).
- You can assign other activities or tasks depending on facilities and equipment.

Cool-Down: 5 Minutes

Select stretching and cool-down activities.

Teaching Tips

A different student from each team can select the fortune fitness task. Assign each team a place to line up and return to after completing tasks. A different person starts in front of the line after completing each task. The activity includes a lot of movement, therefore discuss safety rules.

Lesson 24

Partner Challenge

Goals

- To improve cardiovascular endurance
- To improve muscular strength

Key Concepts

There are many reasons why people are physically inactive. These may include inconvenience of facilities and activities, cost of activities, lack of time, dislike of activity, lack of knowledge about the benefits of physical exercise. However, individuals are likely to participate in activities if they can participate with a friend.

Materials

One ball (per pair of students)

Warm-Up: 5 Minutes

Select stretching and warm-up activities.

Activity: Partner Challenge

- Divide class into pairs.
- Establish and demonstrate a series of partner activities (see fig. 5.1). Some include a ball, others do not.
- Specify the number of repetitions for each student before changing roles.
- Students complete the following:

A. Corner link

Students link elbows with partner and skip to each corner of the playing area in turn. At each corner, students complete one push-up and after visiting each corner, return to the middle.

B. Partner toss

Students face each other lying on stomach. Backs are arched with knees and elbows off the ground. Pass a ball back and forth, one throwing in air, the other rolling ball along ground.

C. Sole pass

One partner tosses the ball to other partner who, lying on his or her back, rebounds it back using the soles of the feet. Bring knees to the chest and thrust legs toward thrower as ball makes contact with the soles of feet.

D. That's using your head

Partners sit facing each other, holding hands while pinching the ball between foreheads. They both stand up, keeping the ball between their foreheads. Then sit back down.

E. Tractor pull

One partner holds the hips of the second partner (while standing behind) and pulls back as the other moves forward. Emphasize that the player is allowed to run but only with a struggle. Switch positions.

F. Mirror movements

One partner moves around copying the running actions of the other partner. Running can be forward, backward, sideways, slow, fast, high, or low.

G. Backing up

Partners sit back to back linking elbows and attempt to stand up.

H. Get a grip

Two partners sit facing one another, each gripping the ball with two hands. Each player leans back and stands up.

Cool-Down: 5 Minutes

Select stretching and cool-down activities.

Teaching Tips

Match partners by size and emphasize safety. Activities are cooperative, not competitive.

WEEK 5

Lesson 25

The Salt Shaker

Goal

- To explain the role of salt in foods and the implications for heart disease

Key Concepts

Salt is a mineral used in food preparation as a flavor enhancer. Most Americans have grown accus-

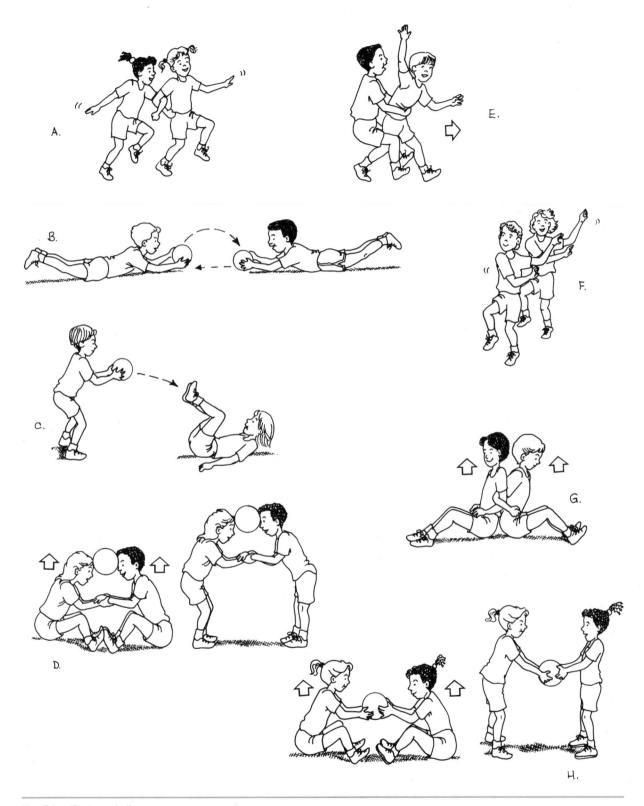

Fig. 5.1.   Partner challenge

tomed to salty tasting foods. It is also used to preserve foods. When used as a preservative, salt attracts water making it unavailable for bacteria to use. Bacteria require water for growth, thus the presence of salt reduces bacterial growth in foods. Table salt is composed of 40 percent sodium and 60 percent chloride. The tongue can sense salty foods. Just as we develop a taste for salt, we can also train our taste buds to adapt to less salty or salt-free foods. For some people, a high-salt diet can increase blood pressure, causing the heart to pump harder and possibly leading to heart disease.

Materials

1. Samples of foods high and low in salt (potato chips, pretzels, salted popcorn, pickles, beef jerky, or salt-free crackers)
2. Salted popcorn marked A
3. Unsalted popcorn marked B
4. Handout 5.2 Week 5, Family Activity: Superstar Veggies and Dip (1 per student)

Activity: The Salt Shaker

- Before class, prepare the food samples by cutting them into bite-sized pieces, enough for the students to sample.
- Clarify the aims of the lesson by discussing the lesson objectives. Ask the students if they know why we put salt on food.
- Identify the role of salt in food—taste and preservation. Show them examples of each, such as ketchup or potato chips for taste, and pickles and beef jerky for preservation.
- Ask the students to recall what the role of salt is to reinforce the concept. Do the students have any experience with salty foods? Do they ever add salt to their food?
- Pass around a sample of a nonsalted food (such as a salt-free cracker). Instruct them to taste the salt-free food and tell them that this food does not have salt added. Then pass out a food that has added salt (such as a saltine cracker). Ask them to taste the food with the salt. Ask them to describe the difference in taste and appearance.
- Next, ask them to taste a salted food (labeled A) without telling them whether salt has been added (popcorn works well). Can they tell whether salt has been added? How? Then give them unsalted sample B. Can they tell the difference?
- Provide samples of preserved foods to taste the salt (beef jerky or pickles). Can they tell by looking at the food whether salt has been added?
- Ask the students to recall the role of salt in foods. Should we worry about the amount of salt we eat each day? Why or why not?
- Strengthen their cognitive responses by asking them what foods they would eliminate if they wanted to reduce the salt in their diet. What other ways could they reduce the salt other than not buying certain foods? (Don't add salt in cooking, or don't add salt to foods at mealtime.)

Handout 5.2   Week 5, Family Activity: Superstar Veggies and Dip

To add color to your diet, try eating fresh vegetables with a low-fat dip.

Ingredients

Fresh vegetables, such as carrots, green pepper, cucumber, celery, mushrooms, cauliflower, broccoli, and cherry tomatoes

Ingredients for dip

2 cups nonfat plain yogurt
2 T. dill weed
2 T. onion powder
2 T. dried parsley leaves
1/2 tsp. paprika
1 tsp. celery seed
(makes 2 cups)

Directions

1. Clean the veggies.
2. Cut into small pieces.
3. Mix dip ingredients.
4. Chill in refrigerator.
5. Serve with veggies.

Time: 20 minutes

Please return by _____.

Week 6: More Aerobic Fitness

The lessons emphasize establishing the difference between aerobic and nonaerobic activities. Further study includes awareness of salt intake and the importance of replacing water lost during exercise.

WEEK 6

Lesson 26

Aerobic Choices

Goals

- To demonstrate activities that are aerobic
- To categorize and graph information

Key Concepts

Every sport or activity has some value because it provides an interest and exercise for students and often increases motivation to be active. However, some sports and activities (such as swimming, running, and bicycling) are better than others for developing heart and lung endurance or cardiovascular fitness. Every student should participate in an activity that promotes cardiovascular fitness.

Materials

Handout 6.1 Aerobic Choices (one per pair)

Activity: Aerobic Choices

Collect and discuss sports cards. Save these for lesson 27. Have children work in pairs. As a fol-low-up to lesson 21, review the basics about aerobic exercise. Remind students that aerobic activities are continuous and make the heart and lungs work hard. Explain that some sports and activities are aerobic in certain aspects. For example, in soccer, players may move continuously for a minute and then may stand still for a while until the ball comes to them. Although children will participate in activities that are fun, they should be encouraged to participate in aerobic activities. An important step in helping children make daily choices in activities is to ask them to determine which activities are aerobic. Use the Aerobic Choices handout and ask students to evaluate each activity. List additional sports for children to assess.

Teaching Tips

Emphasize there are no good or bad activities, but that different activities have varying benefits. Being a pitcher in baseball or a football place kicker requires high levels of skill rather than aerobic fitness.

Handout 6.1   Aerobic Choices

1. Swimming _____

2. Baseball pitcher _____

3. Soccer (field player) _____

4. Watching TV _____

5. Jogging or running _____

6. Basketball _____

7. Bicycling _____

8. Soccer goalie _____

9. Jumping rope _____

10. Football _____

If the listed activities include continuous motion, can be played for 15 to 20 minutes, and use the large muscles of the body, place an A next to the activity (A for aerobic). Write N next to those that are not aerobic. If an activity seems to fall in between, place an AN next to it. After labeling activities, transfer names to Venn diagram (fig. 6.1).

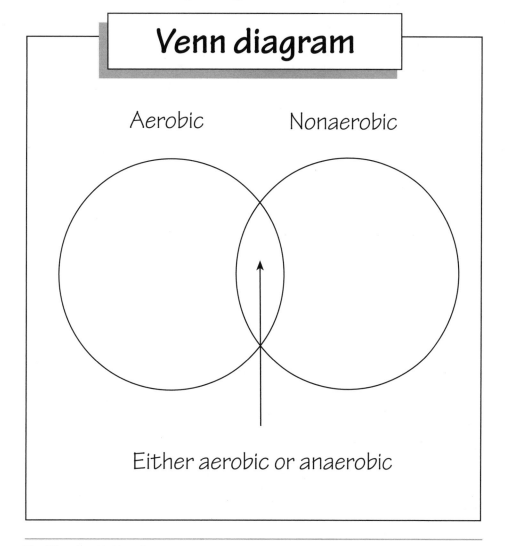

Fig. 6.1.   Aerobic Venn diagram

Lesson 27

Aerobic Voyage

Goals

- To improve cardiovascular fitness
- To help students distinguish between aerobic and nonaerobic activities

Key Concepts

Nonaerobic (or anaerobic is a commonly used term) activities are carried out without oxygen. The intensity of nonaerobic activities is so high that oxygen is not used to produce energy. Because energy production is limited in the absence of oxygen, these activities (e.g., 50-yard sprint) can be done for only short periods. Anaerobic activities contribute little to the development of the cardiovascular system.

Materials

1. Twenty sports cards (from Family Activity)
2. Cones to mark off a large playing area (can be as large as 50 × 50 yards)
3. Pinnies (enough for half your class)

Warm-Up: 5 Minutes

Select stretching and warm-up activities.

Activity: Aerobic Voyage

- Discuss with the class the characteristics of aerobic physical activity.
- Use 20 pictures of activities (sports cards), 10 aerobic and 10 not aerobic in this activity.
- Place five aerobic and five nonaerobic cards in each team's safe area. Place cards on the floor face down (see fig. 6.2)
- Divide the playing area into two halves with cones, then split the class in two with one team in each half.

- Put colored pinnies on one team for identification.
- The objective of the game is for one team to get all aerobic activity cards in their safe area.
- Once players pass over the middle line into the opposing team's territory, they can be tagged and must freeze in that spot. To get unfrozen, a teammate must crawl through their legs. Players cannot be tagged if they make it into the opposing team's safe area.
- They may take one card at a time, and try to run back to their side without being tagged. They can pick up several cards and decide which one to take.
- If tagged, they must release the card to the tagger (who can replace card in own safe area) and freeze where they were tagged.
- If they are not tagged, they return to their own side and place the card in their safe area and try to get another card.
- The safe area can't be guarded. It must remain clear for a six-foot distance.
- Play for a five-minute period and determine which team has the most aerobic cards.

Cool-Down: 5 Minutes

Select stretching and cool-down activities.

Teaching Tips

Laminating the cards before the game will prevent them from being damaged. For aerobic activities use pictures of jogging, bicycling, jump rope, basketball, soccer, dancing, and ice skating. For nonaerobic activities use pictures of football, baseball, shot put, discuss, javelin throw, bowling, golf, and kickball.

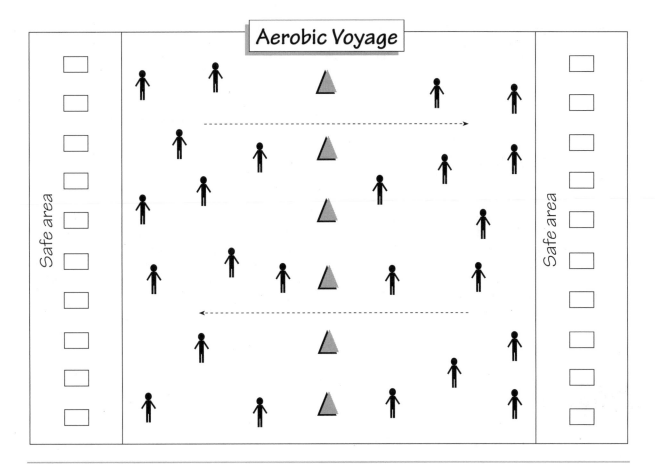

Fig. 6.2. Aerobic voyage

Lesson 28

Sodium Search

Goals

- To improve cardiovascular fitness
- To improve cooperation skills

Key Concepts

About 75 percent of our daily sodium intake comes from processed foods. For example, a serving of canned beans contains approximately 150 milligrams of sodium, whereas the same serving of fresh cooked beans has approximately 5 milligrams. To reduce sodium intake to 1100 milligrams per day, eat fresh foods prepared without added salt.

Materials

1. Five or six paper bags
2. Twenty-five food labels
3. A six-by-nine-inch card and pencil for each group

Warm-Up: 5 Minutes

Select stretching and warm-up activities.

Activity: Sodium Search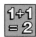

- Review labels ahead of time in class.
- Organize class into teams of five.

- Each team has a bag with a variety of food labels that contain sodium on the list of food ingredients. The back of each label has the name of an exercise written on it.
- Place the bag with labels 30 to 40 yards away from team.
- The first team member runs to their bag and takes out a label and returns to the team.
- Students review the label for sodium content. Students perform exercises (specify exercises from chapter 13) according to the following.
- Third graders add the first two numbers together. For example, if the number of milligrams is 380, second graders add 3 and 8 and complete 11 repetitions.
- Fourth graders add all digits and complete that number of repetitions.
- The team records the name of the food label and the number of milligrams of sodium per serving on its card.
- The next student runs to get a new label.
- The relay continues until all students have retrieved a label. Change labels between teams and repeat.

Cool-Down: 5 Minutes

Select stretching and cool-down activities.

Teaching Tips

During cool-down, discuss those foods that had the highest amounts of sodium. Those foods with 600 milligrams or greater are high in sodium relative to a daily intake of 1100 milligrams. Circle on the food label the section for nutrition information per serving.

WEEK 6

Lesson 29

Carbo Search

Goals

- To improve cardiovascular fitness
- To determine which type of food has the highest amount of carbohydrates

Key Concepts

Carbohydrates provide the major energy source for the body. The major sources of complex carbohydrates are bread, cereals, fruits, and vegetables. Emphasize that a diet high in complex carbohydrates provides the most energy.

Materials

1. Foam balls for taggers
2. Cones

Warm-Up: 5 Minutes

Select stretching and warm-up activities.

Activity: Carbo Search

- Mark two lines with cones 30 yards apart.
- Divide class into three groups, each group representing one of the following foods: steak, milk, and bananas.
- One person is the tagger who stands in the middle of the playing area. The rest of the class lines up on one endline facing the tagger.
- The tagger will begin by calling out either "steak," "milk," or "bananas." Steak means the students have to hop to get across because it is low in carbohydrates. Milk means the students have to skip to get across because it has a moderate amount of carbohydrates, and bananas mean the students have to run across because they have a high amount of carbohydrates.
- Once the students have made it to the other endline without being tagged, they are safe.
- If they are tagged, they become taggers too. Only the initial tagger does the calling.

- The banana group should be able to survive the longest because they can run.

Cool-Down: 5 Minutes

Select stretching and cool-down activities.

Teaching Tips

Make sure the playing area is large enough so students are moving regularly. You could substitute any meat or fish for steak. Yogurt, cheese, or other dairy products could substitute for milk, and any fruit, vegetable, cereal, or bread would substitute for banana.

Lesson 30

Do Yourself a Flavor

WEEK 6

Goals

- To understand the importance of replacing water lost during exercise
- To understand that sweat is the body's mechanism for controlling body temperature

Key Concepts

Exercise can produce large amounts of heat, but if you don't have enough water in your body (a condition called dehydration) you may not be able to exercise effectively. Initially, your heart begins to work harder and your pulse rate increases. You also begin to get tired and can get headaches and become nauseated. These effects reduce your ability to exercise. Thus, the ability to produce sweat is an important body temperature regulatory mechanism. Your body sweats, the air dries your skin, and you feel cooler. Sweat is mostly water—about 75 percent—with the remaining 25 percent being various salts and minerals. It's important, therefore, to replace the water first and allow the salts and minerals to be replenished with food consumed after you exercise. The best way to replace the water you lose during exercise is to drink cool water in combination with a balanced diet, on a day-to-day basis. If you weigh yourself before and after exercise and find that you have lost weight, that weight is mostly water. For every pound of water you lose, you should consume two cups of water. We should drink at least six to eight (eight-ounce) glasses of water each day, plus additional water for sweat loss. Many sports drinks have been developed for exercise. Some drinks contain sugar in the form of glucose or fructose, as well as salts such as potassium, sodium, and magnesium. These drinks are not necessary to replace fluids lost during exercise. Water is more important. You can replace sugar and salt after exercise in the food you eat.

Materials

1. Samples of sports drinks, such as Gatorade, Erg, All Sport, and water, labeled A, B, C, and so forth
2. Handout 6.2 Do Yourself a Flavor (one per pair)
3. Small sample-size paper cups (enough for each student to have one for each sample)
4. Handout 6.3 Week 6, Family Activity: Waterlogged (one per student)

Activity: Do Yourself a Flavor

- Before class, pour the sports drinks into containers marked A, B, C, and so forth. Use the empty drink bottles for the label-reading activity. Also include a bottle of water, such as spring water. You can remove labels from the sports drinks and copy them before the lesson.
- Begin the discussion about sweating. How many students felt their skin after exercise? Was it wet? Was it gritty feeling? If yes, why was it gritty?

- Discuss the importance of water in sweat during exercise and how to replace fluid after exercise.
- Show the students some samples of sports drinks. Have they ever tried them? Did they like them? Why did they drink them? Discuss briefly what the drinks contain.
- Ask the students to work with a partner. Instruct them to read the labels of each of the drinks and record the ingredients on the comparison chart.
- After they have completed the chart, ask the students to sample each drink and rate the taste in a blind test (only you know which drink s A, B, and C are). Can they identify by the taste and by the list of ingredients which drinks are which?
- Discuss with the class which drink had sugar added. What about salts? Which drink did they like the best? How would they compare them to the water? Which would be the most effective to prevent dehydration?

Teaching Tips

An additional activity would include calculating the cost of each drink and evaluating this compared to water.

Handout 6.2   Do Yourself a Flavor

COMPARISON CHART

Sport drink	Ingredients	Sugar (Y/N)	Salt (Y/N)
_____	_____	_____	_____
	_____		
	_____		
	_____		
	_____		
_____	_____	_____	_____
	_____		
	_____		
	_____		
_____	_____	_____	_____
	_____		
	_____		
	_____		

TASTE TEST

Drink	Salty	Sweet	Like it (Y/N)
1. A _____	_____	_____	_____
2. B _____	_____	_____	_____
3. C _____	_____	_____	_____
4. _____	_____	_____	_____
5. _____	_____	_____	_____

Handout 6.3   Week 6, Family Activity: Waterlogged

This is an activity for you and one additional family member. On a weekend day, fill two containers with at least four large glasses of water in each container. Throughout the day when you are thirsty, drink from your individual container. Record in the log the times during the day when you drink. The goal is to drink all four glasses by the next morning. Place this on the fridge door for each reading.

Name_____   Name_____

Drinking times:

Time: 10 minutes

Please return by _____.

Week 7: Flexibility Fitness

Lessons 32, 33, and 34 include a special segment called Flex Focus. They emphasize specific body parts in the warm-up for flexibility training. The purpose of this segment is to teach stretching exercises designed to improve flexibility for specific joints in the body.

WEEK 7

Lesson 31

Winning Warm-Ups

Goals

- To teach the importance of flexibility exercises as part of a warm-up routine
- To emphasize the need for gentle activity before a workout

Key Concepts

Flexibility exercises are an essential part of any warm-up routine. Stretching is a habit that children need to develop as part of a safe approach to rigorous exercise. The goal is to warm up and stretch the entire body; however, emphasize the primary body part(s) used for a specific sport or activity. These movements supply the muscles with extra oxygen and raise the temperature of muscles.

Materials

1. Old sports magazines
2. Additional copies of warm-up and cool-down stretches (chapter 10)
3. Handout 7.1 Warming Up to Win the Workout
4. Handout 7.2 Warming Up to Win the Workout (sample)

Activity: Winning Warm-Ups

Ask your students if they have observed participants at a sporting event. Watch what athletes do before competing. They will observe two things. First, athletes are performing movements in slow motion or at a gentle pace. Baseball players throw the ball back and forth, soccer players pass a ball back and forth, tennis players rally with an opponent, and gymnasts practice approaches to apparatus. Second, stretching exercises are essential in a warm-up routine. Stretching activities loosen up the elastic parts of the body, the muscles, and lower the risk of injuries. The smart exerciser realizes that the best warm-ups for any activity are those that use the motions needed in the activity. Children in groups of three or four can design their own warm-ups. From sports magazines, pick out pictures of an individual involved in a vigorous sport, for example, a cross-country skier, a basketball player, a baseball player, or a tennis player. Use handout 7.1 to help design warm ups. Handout 7.2 is presented as an example. Give special care to stretching those parts of the body used in the sport. Students can draw the exercises on the page or write a description of each activity. Have groups share and demonstrate their winning warm-ups.

Teaching Tips

Emphasize exercise safety and remind students that the cool-down phase is very similar to the warm-up phase.

Handout 7.1   Warming Up to Win the Workout

Sport_____

Primary body parts used in sport

Stretching activities
Describe three specific stretches that stretch the joints used in the sport.

Reduced speed activities
Skill warm-up

Handout 7.2   Warming Up to Win the Workout

Sport <u>Soccer</u>

Primary body part used in sport
Legs

Stretching activities
Describe three specific stretches that stretch the joints used in the sport.
1. Sitting stretch
2. Single leg tuck
3. Calf stretch

Reduced speed activities
Skill warm-up

    1. Passing soccer ball in pairs
    2. Dribbling soccer ball across the field
    3. Shooting at the goal concentrating on accuracy but not power

WEEK 7

Lesson 32

Target Fitness II

Goals

- To improve cardiovascular fitness
- To improve muscular endurance
- To improve shoulder flexibility

Key Concepts

Realization of specific goals in physical fitness fosters a positive outlook toward physical activity. In this lesson students have an opportunity to improve, compare, and revise their goals from lesson 22. Back exercise helps strengthen and increase flexibility in the muscles and joints that support the back.

Materials

1. Mats
2. Target Fitness Sheet from lesson 22
3. New Target Fitness Sheet, Handout 7.3

Warm-Up: 5 Minutes

Select stretching and warm-up activities. Lessons 32, 33, and 34 include a special segment called Flex Focus. It emphasizes specific body parts in the warm-up for flexibility training. The purpose of this segment is to teach stretching exercises to improve flexibility for specific joints in the body, especially the chest and lower back.

Flex Focus: Chest (see fig. 7.1)

1. *Chest stretcher*
   In a prone (lying on stomach) position, lift upper body off the ground so the arms are straight. Complete five times.

2. *Swimmer*
   Tilt the trunk slightly forward. Imitate a freestyle swim stroke. Complete 10 to 12 strokes with each arm.

Flex Focus: Low Back (see fig. 7.1)

1. *Sit and reach*
   Sit with knees slightly bent and feet pointed upward. Reach toward toes. Bend forward from the hips. Try to pull the chin toward the knees. Hold for 10 to 20 seconds. Repeat two or three times.

2. *Back stretcher*
   Pull the right leg toward the chest by holding onto the thigh. Keep the left leg slightly bent. Hold for 20 to 30 seconds. Switch legs. Repeat two or three times.

3. *Pill bug*
   Pull both legs to the chest by holding onto the hamstrings. Curl the head up toward the knees. Hold for 5 to 15 seconds. Repeat two or three times.

Activity: Target Fitness II

In this lesson students repeat the exercises from lesson 22 and aim to reach their goals.

Cool-Down: 5 Minutes

Select stretching and cool-down activities.

Teaching Tips

Conclude this lesson with a discussion about setting goals. Were the goals too easy or difficult? Did setting specific goals motivate them to reach their target? Do they need to adjust up or down? What factors influence performance? What is more important, improvement or reaching goals? Students can write a revised goal for each fitness activity. Some may be on target and simply need to continue workout program. Students can graph their results from Target Fitness I and II and write a paragraph summarizing their performances.

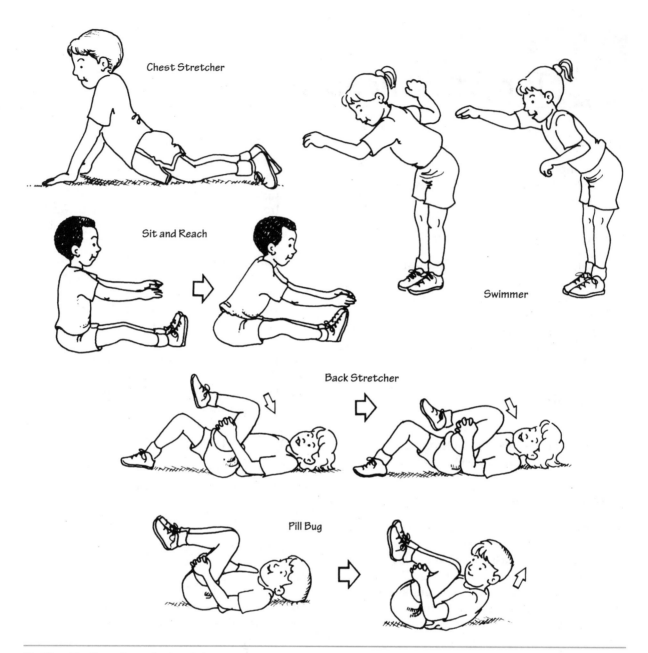

Fig. 7.1.   Flex focus: Lower back and chest

Handout 7.3.   Target Fitness Sheet

Name_____   Date_____

	Previous goal	Number performed	Revised goal 2
Push-ups or modified push-ups	_____	_____	_____
Side leg raises	_____	_____	_____
Mountain climbers	_____	_____	_____
Thigh lifts	_____	_____	_____
Sit-ups	_____	_____	_____
Jumping jacks	_____	_____	_____

WEEK 7

Lesson 33

Turn to Fitness

Goals

- To improve muscular endurance
- To improve cardiovascular fitness
- To improve coordination

Key Concepts

Long rope jumping is an excellent activity for beginning jumpers. Effective turning is the key to successful jumping. Turning the rope is a difficult skill and should be practiced regularly to achieve rhythm.

Materials

Long jump ropes (one per three students is ideal)

Warm-Up: 5 Minutes

Select stretching and warm-up activities. Give special emphasis to the legs.

Flex Focus: Upper Legs (see fig. 7.2)

1. *Sitting stretcher*
   Sit with soles of feet together, legs flat on the floor. Place hands on knees and lean forearms against knees; resist while trying to raise knees. Hold five to seven seconds, then relax.

2. *Hip and thigh stretcher*
   Place right knee directly above right ankle and stretch left leg backward so the knee touches the floor. If necessary, place hands on floor for balance. Press pelvis forward and downward and hold. Repeat on other side.

Flex Focus: Lower Legs (see fig. 7.2)

1. *Calf stretch*
   Stand with right leg forward and left leg back. Keep left leg straight and bend right leg. Lean forward, keeping heel of left foot on ground. Repeat for right leg.

2. *Shin stretcher*
   Kneel on both knees, turn to right, press down on right ankle with right hand and hold. Keep hips thrust forward to avoid hy-

perflexing knees. Do not sit on heels. Repeat on left side.

Activity: Turn to Fitness

- Organize students into groups of three.
- Start by having children practice turning the rope with an even, steady rhythm.
- Children are ready to try long rope jumping when they can jump in place with both feet leaving the ground simultaneously.
- Use the following buildup skills to develop basic jumping skills:
  1. Place long rope on floor and children jump back and forth with small continuous two-foot jumps.
  2. Turners slowly move the rope back and forth along the floor and jumper jumps over it.
  3. The turners move the rope in a pendulum swing while the jumper jumps the rope each time.
  4. Teach front door and back door entry. Front door means the jumper enters from the side where the rope is turning forward. Back door means the jumper enters from the side where the rope is turning backward and away from the jumper.
  5. Turners move rope with a full swing. Jumper stands behind one of the turners and practices jumping every time the rope touches the floor.
- Teach the following activities:
  1. Jumper stands in center between the turners who turn rope over the jumper's head. As the rope completes the turn, the jumper exits.
  2. Run through the turning rope, without jumping and following the rope through.
  3. Jumper stands in center and tries to jump as many times as possible.
  4. Jumper runs to center, and jumps five times.
  5. Jumper stands in center and jumps two times as rope is turned in the one direction, and two times in the opposite direction.

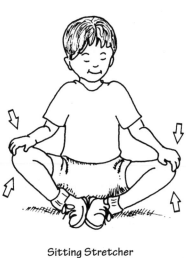

Sitting Stretcher

Hip and Thigh Stretcher

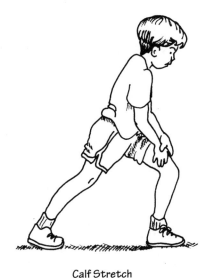

Calf Stretch

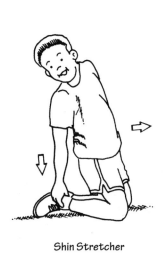

Shin Stretcher

Fig. 7.2. Flex focus: Legs

6. While the rope is being turned, the jumper runs in (front door), jumps once, and runs out.
7. Jumper runs to center, jumps five times, and runs out.
8. Jumper runs to center and jumps five times on right foot only.
9. Jumper runs to center and jumps five times on left foot only.
10. Jumper runs to center and jumps 10 times.

Cool-Down: 5 Minutes

Select stretching and cool-down activities.

Teaching Tips

Rotate children from turners to jumpers regularly. In turning a rope, emphasize the following. Keep elbow close to body and turn rope with forearm. Keep the thumb in an upright position. Hold the rope in front of the body at waist level. Long turning ropes should be between 12 to 18 feet in length. Use three-eighths to five-eighths-inch diameter rope. Your local chapter of the American Heart Association may loan videotapes of jump roping skills.

Lesson 34

Challenge Course

WEEK 7

Goals

- To improve cardiovascular endurance
- To improve locomotor skills
- To improve flexibility of neck and shoulders

Key Concepts

Challenge courses provide an opportunity to practice a variety of movement skills and experience vigorous exercise. Students enjoy negotiating the obstacles and the challenge of completing the course as quickly and accurately as possible. This approach to exercise is often associated with military and adventure physical training.

Materials

1. Ten cones
2. Mats
3. Benches
4. Four to six hoops
5. Six jump ropes
6. Yardstick (for bar)

Warm-Up: 5 Minutes

Select stretching and warm-up activities. Give special emphasis to stretching the neck and shoulder.

Flex Focus: Neck (see fig. 7.3)

1. *Neck stretch*
   Keeping shoulders back and spine straight, slowly roll the head to the left shoulder, straighten, then roll toward right shoulder, straighten. Repeat five times. Do not roll the head in a fast, circular manner or roll head backward.

Flex Focus: Shoulder (see fig. 7.3)

1. *Shoulder shrug (helps to reduce muscle tension in neck and shoulders)*
   Shrug both shoulders up toward your ears. Hold and repeat. Shrug shoulders forward as far as possible. Hold and repeat. Shrug shoulders backward as far as possible. Hold and repeat. Shrug each shoulder opposite ways, up and down. Hold and repeat.

2. *Reach for the stars*
   Hold both hands together and reach above the head.

3. *Shoulder squeeze (stretches back of arms and shoulders)*
   Hold both hands behind your back (standing position). Straighten the arms. Lift the arms up and away from the back. Try not to lean forward (repeat two or three times).

Activity: Challenge Course

- Set up a challenge course in the gym or outdoors.
- The course is a series of obstacles arranged in a circle. The specific nature of the challenge course depends on available facilities and equipment. A sample is shown in fig. 7.4. The course should be wide enough for several students to move around at the same time. Avoid using obstacles that create a line of children who have to wait to use that piece of equipment.
- Demonstrate the specific movements. The objective is to keep moving as quickly as possible on the course.
- The course can include all types of locomotor movements (running, jumping, galloping, hopping), moving under, over, through, and around obstacles, and animal walks or movements.
- Divide class into pairs, with one student completing the course and the other jogging or walking around the outside.
- Partners change after two minutes.

Cool-Down: 5 Minutes

Select stretching and cool-down activities.

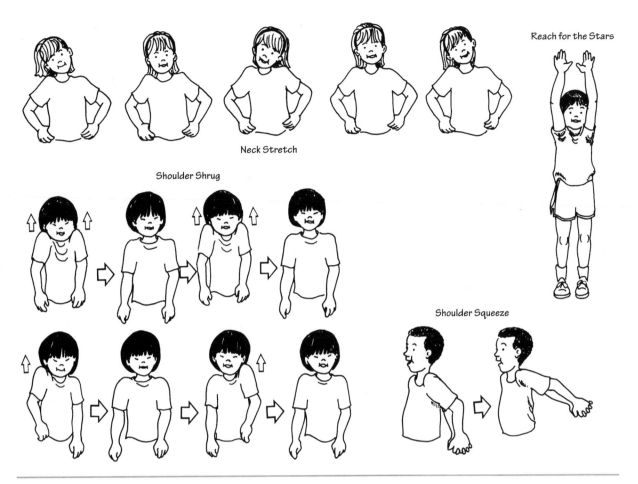

Fig. 7.3. Flex focus: Neck and shoulder

Teaching Tips

Challenge students to keep moving! An alternative format is for each partner to complete two circuits and then change with the other partner. You can use other equipment items, such as chairs, balance beams, inclined mats, climbing ropes, and scooter boards. Use students as station judges to keep equipment organized and assure accuracy of movements.

WEEK 7

Lesson 35

Carbo Loading

Goals

- To establish the importance of eating carbohydrates as part of a healthy diet
- To test which foods contain complex carbohydrates

Key Concepts

To function and grow properly, the human body has certain basic needs that must be met. The most important is the production of energy. Foods that contain carbohydrates are needed by the brain

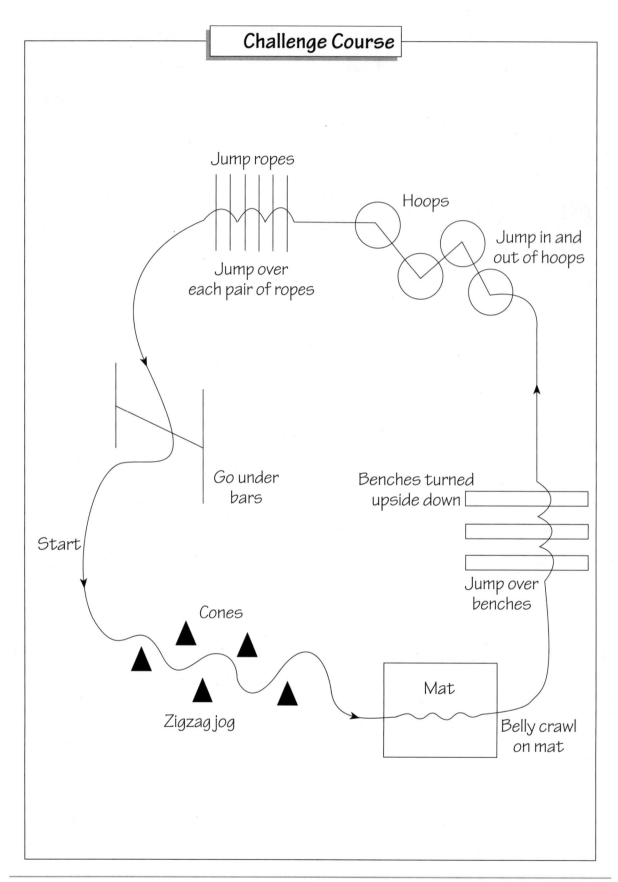

Fig. 7.4.   Challenge course

and muscles for fuel and by the digestive tract to process food and provide roughage. Carbohydrates provide the body with energy to meet a student's daily needs for growth and energy. The foods high in carbohydrates include bread, pasta, fruits, and vegetables. Carbohydrates are the only major nutrient that has not been linked to long-term health warnings. When you place a drop of iodine on a food that contains complex carbohydrates, it turns blue.

Materials (per group)

1. Iodine (clear) mixed with water
2. An eye dropper
3. Newspaper
4. Food samples: saltine crackers, pieces of egg white, pieces of cheese and bologna or other sandwich meat, pieces of meat (e.g., hamburger), boiled white rice, cooked pasta, slices of white bread, and tortillas
5. Handout 7.4 Carbo Loading
6. Handout 7.5 Week 7, Family Activity: Family Triathlon (one per student)

Activity: Carbo Loading

- Ask the students how they feel after not eating for a long time. Do they feel tired? What foods do they think might provide more energy than others? Write answers on the board.
- Review the information presented in the key concepts with the class.
- Organize the class into small groups. Using the food samples, ask the groups to categorize the foods by food groups, and write them on their handout. Demonstrate with one food item how complex carbohydrates turn blue when iodine is applied. Ask the students to predict which of the remaining foods contain complex carbohydrates.
- Give each group a newspaper, samples of foods, and the iodine solution. Instruct the students to put a drop of the iodine solution on each sample with an eye dropper. Record on the handout what happens to the food. Complex carbohydrates in the form of starch will turn blue.
- As a class, discuss their findings. How did their results compare to their predictions? Relate their findings to their past experience.

Handout 7.4   Carbo Loading

Samples	Food group or category	Prediction (Y/N)	Results (Y/N)
1. _____	_____	_____	_____
2. _____	_____	_____	_____
3. _____	_____	_____	_____
4. _____	_____	_____	_____
5. _____	_____	_____	_____
6. _____	_____	_____	_____
7. _____	_____	_____	_____
8. _____	_____	_____	_____

Describe your observations. (Do certain categories of foods change color and others don't?)

Handout 7.5   Week 7, Family Activity: Family Triathlon

A triathlon consists of running, swimming, and bicycling. Triathletes are outstanding endurance athletes. Take the triathlon concept and have fun with your family. Choose three activities that your family enjoys, such as walking, bicycling, jogging, jumping rope, soccer, basketball, touch football, or others. Select the three sports or activities to do one after the other for a total of 30 minutes. One activity may last longer than others. Discuss your results of the triathlon in class. Write a paragraph about your Family Triathlon.

Time: 30 minutes

Please return by _____.

CHAPTER

8

Week 8: Strength Fitness

Lessons 37, 38, and 39 include a special segment called Muscle Moment. They emphasize specific body parts after the warm-up for strength training. The purpose of this segment is to teach exercises to increase strength of specific areas of the body.

WEEK 8

Lesson 36

The Big Ten

Goal

- To help children identify the names and locations of 10 major muscle groups

Key Concepts

There are more than 600 muscles in the body and the major muscles are shown in fig. 8.1. Most muscles in the human body have Greek or Latin names (deltoids, pectorals, biceps). Children are more likely to understand muscle function and development if they know the names and locations of the muscles used in specific exercises.

Materials

1. Masking tape and pens
2. Diagram of major muscle groups, one per pair

Activity: The Big Ten

Use the diagram of the body muscle groups (fig. 8.1) to help children locate the Big Ten. Divide class into pairs and give each pair masking tape and a pen. Using pieces of masking tape, help children tape the names of the major muscle groups on each other. Help children identify and locate the following: biceps, triceps, quadriceps, hamstrings, deltoids, calves, abdominals, latissimus dorsi, pectorals, and trapezius.

Teaching Tips

Demonstrate with one child or another adult the procedure of putting the name on the correct muscle location. Children of the same gender should pair up. Use slang names for muscles, bi's (biceps), tri's (triceps), quads (quadriceps), delts (deltoids), calf (calves), hams (hamstrings), lats (latissimus dorsi), pecs (pectorals), and traps (trapezius).

Dr. Simon Says: Play the typical Simon says game but use names and locations of muscles. When student is out have them perform an exercise using that muscle, then rejoin the game.

WEEK 8

Lesson 37

Soccer 3

Goals

- To improve the strength of triceps, biceps, and deltoid muscles
- To improve cardiovascular fitness
- To improve soccer skills

Key Concepts

You can modify traditional team sports to increase participation and activity. Reducing the number of players on each team guarantees full participation and a more active game. Children get to touch the ball more often and this promotes skill development.

Materials

1. Two soccer balls
2. Eight cones
3. Pinnies

Warm-Up: 5 Minutes

Select stretching and warm-up activities. The Muscle Moment features a specific body part and

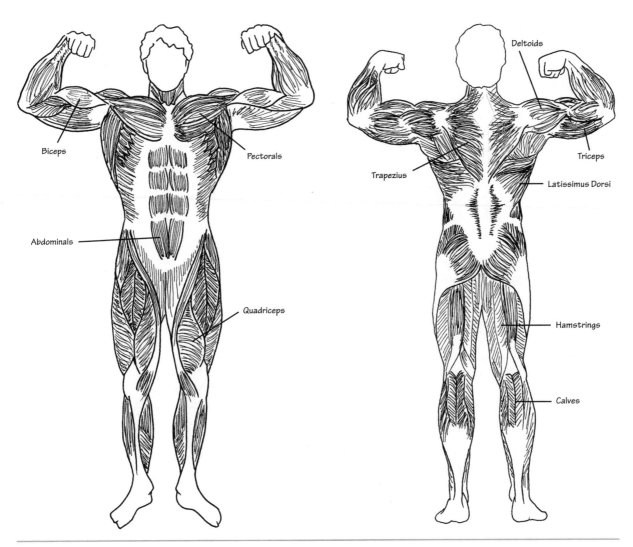

Fig. 8.1.   *The muscular system*

provides exercises to strengthen that part. Give special emphasis to the arms, shoulders, and chest following the warm-up (see fig. 8.2).

Muscle Moment: Arms and Shoulders

The triceps muscle is on the back of the upper arm. The push-up uses the triceps muscle to help lift you off the floor. The biceps muscle is on the front of the upper arm and allows you to curl your arm and bend your elbow. As you eat food, the biceps muscle allows you to move the fork to your mouth. The deltoid muscle is located on top of the shoulder and lifts the arm at the shoulder. The deltoid muscle helps lift objects and helps in throwing. Complete the following to strengthen these three muscles. See chapter 13 for exercise descriptions.

1. *Side standers*
   Student lies in prone position with chest touching floor, legs and feet together. Hands are directly under shoulders. Raise body in push-up fashion. At full arm extension, rotate body one-quarter turn to left, supporting weight on right hand and foot. Return to starting position. Rotate body to the right, supporting weight on the left hand and foot. Return to starting position.

2. *Crab legs*
   Start in a crab position. Support weight on hands and feet. Extend right leg forward. Extend left leg as right leg is brought back. Return to starting position.

3. *Crab walkers*
   Start in a crab position. Support weight on

hands and feet. Move right hand and left foot forward simultaneously. Move left hand and right foot forward simultaneously.

Muscle Moment: Chest

The main chest muscles are the pectorals. The pectorals are shaped like a fan and help to cover and protect the upper ribs. The pectorals help you pull the arm across the front of the body. They are used in hugging.

1. *Push-ups or modified push-ups*
   Lie on stomach with chest touching the floor and feet together. Hands are under the shoulders. Push and raise body by extending arms. Raise body in straight line, not allowing back to sway. Lower body until chin touches ground. For a modified push-up the knees are resting on the floor.

Activity: Soccer 3

- Divide class into groups of six.
- Mark out two playing areas 40 × 40 yards as shown in fig. 8.2.
- Two teams play against each other with three players from each team acting as goalkeepers.
- The remaining three players try to score in the opponent's goal.
- Change goalkeepers and players every two minutes.
- If ball goes out of play over the sidelines, players throw ball back into play using soccer throw-in.

Cool-Down: 5 Minutes

Select stretching and cool-down activities.

Teaching Tips

Children can play this activity on the field or playground. Use a low inflated ball on the play-

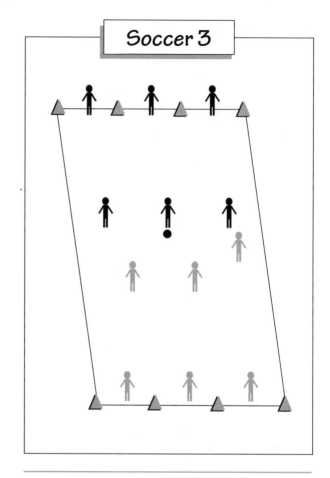

Fig. 8.2.   Soccer 3

ground to prevent ball bouncing too much or rolling away when out of bounds. If there is an odd number of players some groups can play 2 versus 2, or 2 versus 3.

WEEK 8

Lesson 38

Jump Rope Kickball

Goals

- To improve cardiovascular fitness
- To improve coordination
- To improve jump rope skills
- To improve the strength of abdominals and back muscles

Key Concepts

This activity combines traditional kickball with jump rope, providing a more active format. Both batting and fielding teams are working cooperatively.

Materials

1. Jump rope for each student
2. Bases
3. Rubber ball
4. Mats

Warm-Up: 5 Minutes

Select stretching and warm-up activities. Emphasize the abdominals and back following the warm-up (see fig. 8.4).

Muscle Moment: Abdominals

The rectus abdominis (abdominals) support and protect body organs. The abdominals allow you to move your spine. Demonstrate four exercises that strengthen the abdominal muscles. Encourage children to start with five repetitions of each exercise. See chapter 13 for exercise descriptions.

1. *Crunches*
   Student lies on floor, legs together, knees bent, and hands across chest. Bring knees and elbows together. Return to starting position.

2. *Bridge backs*
   Student is on hands and knees in crawling position with feet shoulder-width apart. Tighten abdominal muscles and arch back as high as possible. Return to starting position. Emphasize importance of tightening abdominal muscles (students should feel it).

3. *Reverse sit-ups (works lower portion of abdomen)*
   Lie on back with bent legs together and arms and hands extended over head. Bend at the waist bringing knees as close to the chest as possible.

4. *Obliques (strengthens side torso)*
   Lie on back with knees bent, feet on floor with hands held lightly behind head. Lift shoulder and upper torso off the floor twisting toward opposite knee. Do not pull head and neck with hands. Return to starting position and repeat on other side. Press spine to floor so hips do not roll.

Muscle Moment: Back

The latissimus dorsi (shortened to lats) are triangle shaped and extend from under the shoulders to the lower back. Lift your right arm over your head and place your left hand under your right shoulder. Slowly pull your right elbow to your right hip and feel your lats muscle contract. The lats help you climb a rope. The trapezius is located on the upper back below the neck and lifts the shoulders up and down as in a shoulder shrug.

1. *Curl-ups*
   In this exercise the lower back acts as a stabilizer. Lie on floor with hands on upper thighs, reach up until upper back comes off the ground.

2. *Chest Raises*
   In this activity the lower back is a prime mover. Lie on stomach with arms at sides and raise chest and head from the ground.

Activity: Jump Rope Kickball

- Divide your class into two teams, batting and fielding. Subdivide the batting team into three squads.
- The first player of the first squad kicks a stationary ball into fair ground.
- The first squad uses jump ropes to go around the bases. Only one player bats at a time from each squad.
- The fielding team collects the ball. Each fielding player has to complete 10 jumps before the fielding player who collected the ball runs in to touch home plate and before the first batting squad reaches home plate.
- After the first squad has run, the second squad is up to bat.
- When all three squads have had one turn, change the teams from fielding to batting.

Cool-Down: 5 Minutes

Select stretching and cool-down activities.

Teaching Tips

The team running base paths has right of way. Younger students unable to jump rope can swing the rope by their side as they run. Make sure there is plenty of space between squad members. Fielding players cannot start their jumps until a fielding player has collected the ball.

WEEK 8

Lesson 39

Terminator Challenge

Goals

- To improve cardiovascular fitness
- To improve strength of calf, hamstring, and quadriceps muscles

Key Concepts

Recent approaches to physical fitness development include cross-training. This uses a variety of activities to develop muscular strength and cardiovascular endurance.

Materials

1. Jump ropes (one per student)
2. Tumbling mats
3. Clipboard with list of student names
4. Stopwatch

Warm-Up: 5 Minutes

Select stretching and warm-up activities. Special emphasis is given to the legs (see fig. 8.5).

Muscle Moment: Upper Legs
The hamstrings are the muscles on the back of the top part of your leg. The hamstrings allow you to bend the knee. Any running activity will use the hamstring muscles. The thigh muscles are one of the strongest muscle groups in the body. The quadriceps are on the front part of the upper leg. Quad means four and there are four long muscles that start near the hip and extend down to the knee. The quadriceps help you straighten your leg. The following exercises use the quadriceps and hamstring muscle groups (in addition to others). Demonstrate the two exercises designed to strengthen the upper legs. Complete 15 repetitions of each. See chapter 13 for exercise descriptions.

1. *Stride jumps*
   Stand with feet together. Jump off ground so feet are spread about three feet apart. Then return to starting position. Similar to jumping jacks with no arm movements.

2. *Leg extensions*
   Kneel on the floor and place hands in front of body. Extend leg behind body and lift.

Muscle Moment: Lower Leg
The calf muscle (gastrocnemius) lifts the foot up and down and helps you stand on your toes and balance. The following exercises use the lower leg.

1. *Heel lifts*
   Stand with feet together. Lift heels off the ground, bend knees slightly, and push off toes into an upright position. Knees should not go past a 90-degree angle. Complete 10 repetitions.

2. *Ten jumps higher*
   Make a series of 10 jumps, each one higher than the previous one. Complete three repetitions.

3. *Sprint starts*
   Start on all fours with right knee forward in a sprinter's stance. On command "set" students raise knees off the ground. On command "go" students run for 10 yards. Complete three repetitions.

Activity: Terminator Challenge

- The students will be timed as to how fast they can accurately perform four tasks: two laps around the field or playground, 50 sit-ups, 100 jumps with a jump rope (jump rope continues despite misses or rests), and 20 push-ups (standard or modified).
- The students begin with the run.
- When finished, they go to the tumbling mats and do 50 sit-ups.
- Then, the students get a rope and complete 100 jumps. Next is 20 push-ups.
- When they are finished, they run to a finish line.

Cool-Down: 5 Minutes

Select stretching and cool-down activities.

Teaching Tips

Students can pair up with partners. While one student is doing his or her activities, the other keeps time. This can be a regular activity for your class. Record scores and challenge children to beat their time in a future Terminator Challenge. A further option is for students in pairs to complete two each of the four tasks. You can also set up Terminator Challenge in a station format with students rotating between activities.

WEEK 8

Lesson 40

From the Label to the Table

Goals

- To read the fat content on the labels of packaged foods
- To reinforce the skill of ordering or grouping foods

Key Concepts

Each prepackaged food provides a nutrition label that you can use to make heart-healthy food choices. Nutrition labels give us a great deal of information about the packaged product. For example, how much fat the food contains per serving is listed in grams. Learning to read and analyze the fat content of packaged foods can help reduce the amount of fat you eat each day. When buying a packaged product, choose products that are either fat free (less than one gram of fat per serving) or low in fat (three grams or less in most cases).

Materials

1. Three kinds of cereal boxes, such as Cheerios or granola
2. Three snack packages, such as potato chips, pretzels, and peanuts
3. Three dessert packages such as cookies, granola bars, and fruit roll-ups
4. Handout 8.1 From the Label to the Table
5. Handout 8.2 Week 8, Family Activity: Label Search (one per student)

Activity: From the Label to the Table

- Before the lesson, set out the packages that the students will investigate. Tell the students that some of these foods may contain fat. Recall from previous lessons that we should reduce fat in our diet. Ask students to predict the item that contains the most fat. Discuss with a partner which one is highest or lowest in fat. Invite students to predict the order of the different groups from the lowest fat content to the highest.
- Explore with the students how they might find out which one has fat and how much fat there is in the food per serving. Using one of the labels, show the students where to find the fat content on the label and how to read it.
- Organize the class into groups of two or three and give each group handout 8.1 From the Label to the Table. Instruct them to read each of the cereal, snack food, and dessert labels provided by the teacher. Record the name of the food and the amount of fat in grams per serving on the handout.
- Next, order all the foods from the least amount of fat to the greatest amount of fat per serving.
- Have students analyze and discuss their results with the class.

Teaching Tips

Before photocopying the handout, write in the names of the foods you've chosen for the lesson. Xerox each food item label for each group or devise a rotation schedule for foods to be passed from group to group.

Handout 8.1   From the Label to the Table

Food	Fat (in grams)	Rank (1 = highest)
Cereals		
1. _____	_____	_____
2. _____	_____	_____
3. _____	_____	_____
Snacks		
1. _____	_____	_____
2. _____	_____	_____
3. _____	_____	_____
Desserts		
1. _____	_____	_____
2. _____	_____	_____
3. _____	_____	_____

Handout 8.2   Week 8, Family Activity: Label Search

Choose six packaged or canned foods from your cupboard. Write down the amount of fat in grams per serving for each food you choose. Then ask your parents if they can place the food in order (from highest to lowest in fat content) without looking at the labels. After they have finished ranking the foods, check to see how many they have right. Switch roles with your parents the second time around, using different foods. Write down the foods and their fat content below. Discuss the results with regard to planning family menu and shopping lists.

PARENT

Food	Prediction	Fat in grams (per serving)	Ranking
1. _____	_____	_____	_____
2. _____	_____	_____	_____
3. _____	_____	_____	_____
4. _____	_____	_____	_____
5. _____	_____	_____	_____
6. _____	_____	_____	_____

STUDENT

Food	Prediction	Fat in grams (per serving)	Ranking
1. _____	_____	_____	_____
2. _____	_____	_____	_____
3. _____	_____	_____	_____
4. _____	_____	_____	_____
5. _____	_____	_____	_____
6. _____	_____	_____	_____

Time: 30 minutes

Please return by_____ .

CHAPTER 9

Week 9: Healthy Lifestyle

The final week focuses on developing personal skills to maintain an active lifestyle. The lessons develop social support strategies in exercise and examine making wise food choices in nutrition.

Lesson 41

Ways to Praise

Goals

- To develop social skills that support exercise
- To reinforce the value of peer support

Key Concepts

Developing a workout plan helps establish an active lifestyle. Selecting appropriate activities that lead to regular exercise and developing ways to motivate and reward each other are essential for sustained participation. It's easier to stick to a program if you know you've got some support.

Materials

Samples of award certificates

Activity: Ways to Praise

Divide class into groups of four. Groups create their own active physical education lesson, including warm-up, activity, and cool-down. In the activity or workout section of the lesson, students develop challenging activities that their classmates can complete. For example, the activity could include 10 push-ups, 15 sit-ups, jog/walk 2 laps or 1/4 mile, 10 jump ropes, dribble 5 lengths of the gym with a basketball. The workout content should be something they can continue individually or with friends. Groups can create their own award certificate to reward individuals who complete their workout. Encourage them to design a fitness logo or seal on the certificate. Ask students to develop five phrases that they can use to motivate and encourage others who participate in exercise. Phrases should support participation, such as, "way to hang in there," or "good effort."

Teaching Tips

Teachers can design a basic certificate that students can complete or use as a model. The praise phrases could be shared orally and teacher can post a list to use in physical education classes. Students can write positive comments about other students and place them in a box or bag. The students should compose them at the beginning of each class session. The teacher can pull four or five slips out and read them aloud (see example below). The students should not sign them.

Dear Mark,

I like the way you always try to do your best and encourage others.

A Healthy Classmate

WEEK 9

Lesson 42

Throw in the Towel

Goals

- To improve strength and endurance
- To reinforce cooperative teamwork

Key Concepts

Exercise is for everyone. Its benefits do not require athletic fitness levels, and all of us can achieve them. Exercise is often associated with competitive sports. The notion that only athletes can achieve physical fitness is false.

Materials

1. Six to eight blankets, beach towels, or old sheets
2. Four volleyballs or soft rubber balls
3. Eight to ten cones

Warm-Up: 5 Minutes

Select stretching and warm-up activities.

Activity: Throw in the Towel

- Divide the class into groups of four.
- Give each group a blanket or large towel.
- Two groups play on opposite sides of a line.
- Use cones to create courts that are 7 or 8 yards wide and 10 yards long.
- The object of the game is to pass the ball the greatest number of consecutive times without the ball touching the ground.
- Players catch the ball in the blanket and toss it to the other team across the line. The ball should only stay in the blanket for three seconds. Teams may initially need to practice moving together.
- When the ball touches the ground, both teams complete an exercise selected from chapter 13.
- Teams count the number out loud as they successfully pass the ball.

Cool-Down: 5 Minutes

Select stretching and cool-down activities.

Teaching Tips

Alternatively, you can set up the activity using a volleyball net and court and the children can keep score. Two blanket teams can play on each side. Give each team their own ball, and teams keep track of the number of consecutive touches and see how high they can make the ball go.

WEEK 9

Lesson 43

Aerobic Kickball

Goals

- To improve cardiovascular fitness
- To improve kicking and catching skills

Key Concepts

Kickball is one of the most popular elementary school physical education activities, however it is inactive. You can modify traditional kickball to provide more activity (running) and increased contact with the ball for all class members.

Materials

1. Four cones or bases
2. One ball

Warm-Up: 5 Minutes

Select stretching and warm-up activities.

Activity: Aerobic Kickball

- Divide the class into two teams.
- Divide the batting team into three groups, A, B, and C. The fielding team spreads out in the field.
- One member of batting group A is up to bat and kicks a stationary ball into the field. All of batting group A run around all the bases.
- A fielder collects the ball and runs to the pitching mound. Everyone else on the fielding team runs to line up behind the player with the ball, and the ball is passed back over the heads of the fielding team.
- The batting group A has to reach home plate before the ball reaches the back person of the fielding team.
- A member of each batting group (A, B, and C) has a turn. Then the fielding and batting teams switch places.

Cool-Down: 5 Minutes

Select stretching and cool-down activities.

Teaching Tips

If students are used to traditional kickball, they may question this new version. Emphasize that in traditional kickball, there is a lot of standing around. This new game provides a lot more activity and involvement. Encourage cooperative and supportive behaviors. The activities of the fielders can be varied. Students can form a circle around the pitcher's mound and pass the ball around the circle. You can increase the distance between the bases so students run farther. Members of the kicking team should remain in order and not pass one another. The kicking team has the right of way on the field.

WEEK 9

Lesson 44

Cardio Cards

Goals

- To improve cardiovascular endurance
- To practice specific exercises to improve muscular strength and endurance

Key Concepts

Leading an active life is so important that it's worth trying different strategies to motivate children to exercise. Use music if it inspires them to exercise. Incorporate discussions of exercise into other curriculum areas. Most important, remember that exercise is not just for the athletically gifted. It is for everyone.

Materials

1. Four cones
2. Index cards with names of exercises (see chapter 13)

3. Sports cards (from Week 4, Family Activity)
4. A deck of cards

Warm-Up: 5 Minutes

Select stretching and warm-up activities.

Activity: Cardio Cards

- Set up four cones to make a square area, 40 × 40 yards or larger, for students to jog around.
- As they pass you, hand out a card with the name of an exercise written on it. Each time they pass you, they trade the card for another.
- At designated intervals, blow a whistle and everyone has to complete the exercise on their card.
- Students complete the number of repetitions according to the number of the playing card drawn by the teacher.

- Include a few sports cards and students have to move around the square imitating actions associated with that game. If students have sports cards they keep moving while others are exercising.

Cool-Down: 5 Minutes

Select stretching and cool-down activities.

Teaching Tips

Students can dribble a basketball or soccer ball around the square and trade it in. Another person handing out and trading cards helps. Emphasize efficient running technique (see lesson 3).

WEEK 9

Lesson 45

Supermarket Sweep

Goals

- To practice reading labels in a grocery store
- To locate and investigate foods in the grocery store with the highest and lowest fat and sodium (salt) content

Key Concepts

Processed foods contain varying amounts of fats and salt, even within the same category of foods (such as crackers and dairy products). For example, you might find crackers ranging from zero to six grams of fat per serving. Learning to read the labels to make wise food choices is important to heart-healthy eating.

Materials

1. Handout 9.1 Supermarket Sweep (one per group)
2. Pencils (one per group)
3. Clipboard (one per group)
4. Handout 9.2 Week 9, Family Activity: Family Fitness Survey (one per student)
5. Handout 9.3 Week 9, Family Activity: Plan of Activity

Activity: Supermarket Sweep

- Explain to the students the objectives of today's lesson.

- Discuss your expectations for their behavior while on a field trip and for the lesson itself.
- Organize the class into six investigative groups as follows:
  1. Crackers and chips group
  2. Dairy group (milk, cheese, and yogurt)
  3. Frozen entree group
  4. Processed meats group
  5. Cereal group
  6. Dessert group (cookies, ice cream, and cake)
- Start with a tour by the store manager. Once the tour has been completed, instruct the students to find their food group aisle and record the aisle number on their handout.
- For the activity, instruct each group to read as many labels as possible and record the food and the amount of fat (in grams) and sodium (in milligrams) per serving for this food. Once they have located a variety of food products, rank them from the highest to the lowest fat and sodium content. Challenge them to find the greatest range of fat and sodium in their food products.

Teaching Tips

Each group should have an adult (parent volunteers) to oversee the process.

Handout 9.1   Supermarket Sweep

Food category_____   Aisle_____

Foods	Grams of fat	Milligrams of sodium	Ranking
_____	_____	_____	_____
_____	_____	_____	_____
_____	_____	_____	_____
_____	_____	_____	_____
_____	_____	_____	_____
_____	_____	_____	_____
_____	_____	_____	_____
_____	_____	_____	_____
_____	_____	_____	_____
_____	_____	_____	_____
_____	_____	_____	_____

Handout 9.2   Week 9, Family Activity: Family Fitness Survey

Make a list of physical fitness activities. Arrange those activities on a piece of paper. Family members can review the list of activities and complete the survey. Use the survey as a way for children and parents to learn more about the interests of family members.

Family member	Activity	Participate in now	Have participated in	Reason why do not participate	Would like to learn
_____	_____	_____	_____	_____	_____
_____	_____	_____	_____	_____	_____
_____	_____	_____	_____	_____	_____
_____	_____	_____	_____	_____	_____
_____	_____	_____	_____	_____	_____
_____	_____	_____	_____	_____	_____
_____	_____	_____	_____	_____	_____
_____	_____	_____	_____	_____	_____

Questions for discussion at home and in class.

1. Are there any similarities in the exercise habits of your family?

2. Do any members of the family exercise or participate together? If so, what activities?

3. Are some members more active than others?

4. Do family members support participation of each other by using phrases such as "good job" or "way to hang in there"?

5. Select one or more activities that the whole family can participate in. Devise a plan or schedule for the family, using the "Plan of Activity."

Time: 25 minutes

Please return by_____.

Handout 9.3   Week 9, Family Activity: Plan of Activity

Family name:

1. Activity:

   Date: Duration:

2. Activity:

   Date: Duration:

3. Activity:

   Date: Duration:

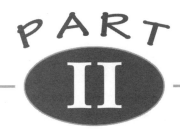

Lesson Elements

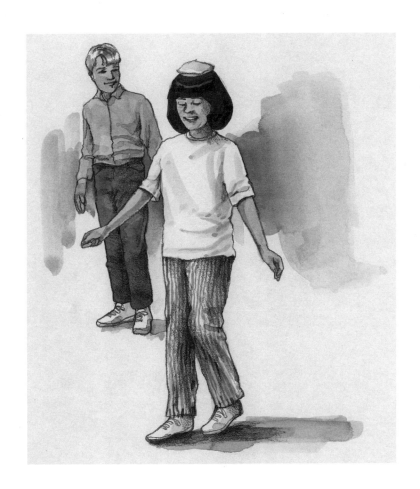

Stretching Routines

Routine 1

For use on the playground (outside) where students cannot lie on the ground (see fig. 10.1).

A. Neck

Keeping shoulders back and spine straight, slowly roll the head to the left shoulder, straighten; then roll toward right shoulder, straighten. Repeat five times. Do not roll head in a fast, circular manner or roll head backward.

B. Back stretch (shoulder and upper arm)

Lift right arm and reach behind head and down the spine. With left hand, push down on right elbow and hold. Reverse arm position and repeat.

C. Side bender (side of body)

Stretch left arm overhead to right. Bend to right at waist, reaching as far to right as possible with the left arm; reach as far as possible to the left with right arm, hold. Repeat on opposite side.

D. Knee pumps (back of upper leg)

While standing, hold the left leg behind the knee and draw it toward your chest. Hold 10 seconds, switch legs, and repeat three times.

E. Heel and toe raise (calf muscles)

Stand with feet close together, hands on hips. Raise up on toes, then heels. Repeat three times.

F. Hip circles (stomach and low back)

Keeping feet and head still, slowly rotate the hips in a sweeping circular motion to loosen the midsection. Repeat 10 times and change direction.

Routine 2

For use inside a gym, multipurpose room, or classroom where students can lie on the floor to stretch (see fig. 10.2).

A. Neck

Keeping shoulders back and spine straight, slowly roll the head to the left shoulder, straighten; then roll toward right shoulder, straighten. Repeat five times. Do not roll head in fast, circular manner or roll head backward.

B. Knee to nose touch (legs and stomach)

In an all fours position, lift the knee to touch the nose. Move the leg back so the leg does not lift higher than the hips, and the neck and lower back are not hyperextended.

C. Shin stretcher (shins)

Kneel on both knees, turn to right and press down on right ankle with right hand and hold. Keep hips thrust forward to avoid hyperflexing knees. Do not sit on heels. Repeat on left side.

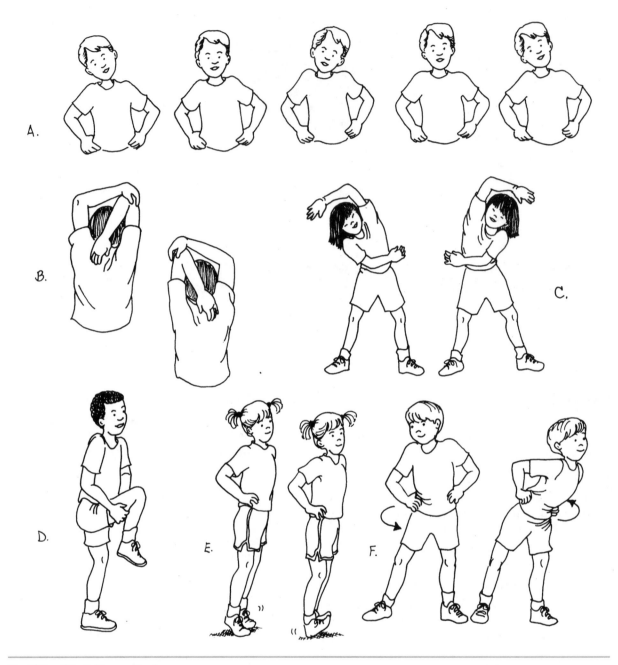

Fig. 10.1.   Stretching routine 1

D. Single leg tuck (back of leg and lower back)

Sit on floor with left leg straight. Tuck right foot against left thigh. Lower chest toward left knee. Repeat with right leg.

E. Low-back stretch (lower back)

Lie on back, and tuck knees to chest.

Routine 3

For use inside a gym, multipurpose room, or classroom where students can lie on the floor to stretch (see fig. 10.3) .

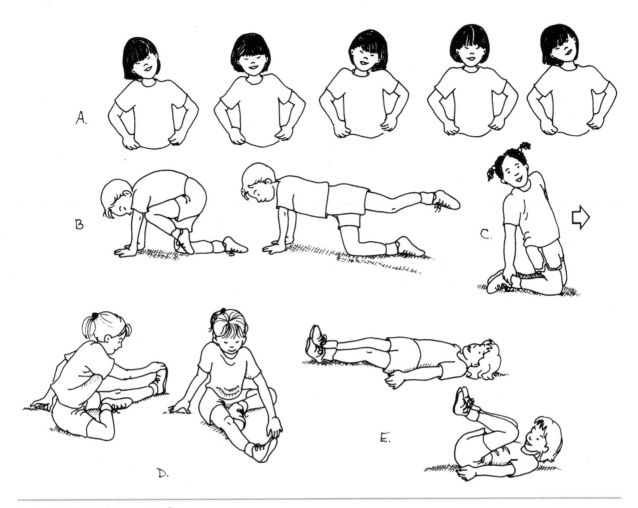

Fig. 10.2. *Stretching routine 2*

A. Sitting stretch (inside of thighs)

Sit with soles of feet together, place hands on knees or ankles, and lean forearms against knees. Resist while attempting to raise knees.

B. Behind neck grasp (back of arms)

Lift right arm and reach behind head and down the spine. With the left hand, reach behind back and grasp the right hand. Reverse hands.

C. One leg stretcher (lower back and back of legs)

Stand with one foot on a bench, keeping both legs straight. Press down on bench with the heel for several seconds; then relax and bend the trunk forward, trying to touch the head to the knee. Hold for a few seconds. Return to starting posi-

tion and repeat with opposite leg. As flexibility increases, the arms can pull the chest toward the legs. Do not lock knee.

D. Arm stretcher (arms and chest)

Cross arms and turn palms of hands together. Raise arms overhead behind ears. Extend at the elbows. Reach as high as possible.

E. Trunk twister (trunk muscles)

Sit with right leg extended, left leg bent and crossed over right knee. Place right arm on the left side of the left leg, and push against that leg while turning the trunk as far as possible to the left. Place left hand on floor behind buttocks. Reverse position and repeat on opposite side.

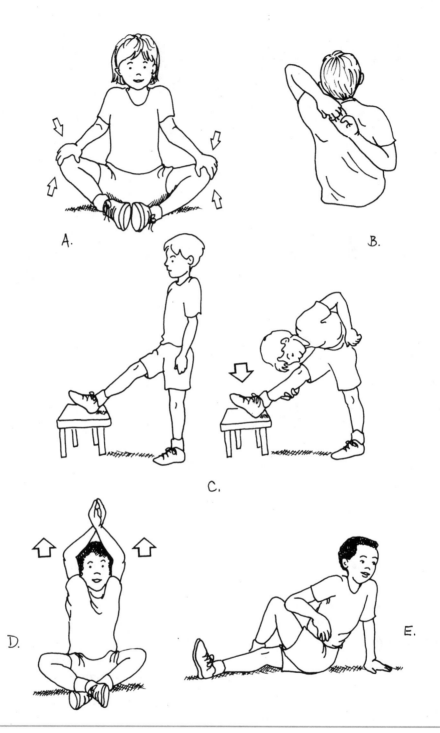

Fig. 10.3.   Stretching routine 3

Warm-Up Activities

Select warm-ups that allow easy transition to the main activity of lesson. For example, the first warm-up would be ideal if the main focus of the lesson is jumping rope. The equipment is already available.

Jump rope and stretch

One rope per student. Each student has jump rope and slowly starts jumping. On signal, the student performs a stretch using the jump rope. An example would be to fold the rope in half and hold it overhead while bending from side to side and to the toes.

Ready, draw!

With partners, each player starts with hands behind their backs. On "Draw," the players show either one or two fingers. If the players show different numbers, they do 10 repetitions of an exercise, for example, jumping jacks. If they show the same numbers, they do nothing and "Draw" again.

Line jump

Students stand next to a line on the playground or in the gym. They jump from side to side without touching the line for 30 seconds. How many times did you cross the line? Try again to see if your score improves on a second attempt.

Triangle tag

In groups of four, two students face each other

and hold hands. The other two stand on either side of the students holding hands. One person is "it" and is chased by the other. The two holding hands act as a shield to the one being chased.

Fifteen-second gusto

15 seconds of jumping jacks
15 seconds of sit-ups
15 seconds of line jumps
15 seconds of jogging on the spot bringing knees up high
15 seconds of modified push-ups

Court line tag

Students play on a basketball court, scattering anywhere on lines. All tags are made below the shoulder with Nerf balls. The two taggers, who tag with Nerf balls, start in the center. During game, players must stay on lines. If tagged, a player takes Nerf ball and immediately becomes a new tagger. Original tagger cannot be immediately tagged.

Kanga ball

In groups of three, two partners face each other and roll a ball back and forth. The third child stands between the pair and jumps over the ball, but turns to keep an eye on it. Roll the ball slowly at first. The objective is not to hit the player in the middle, but to make the player jump. Players can kick the ball back and forth or sit with their legs spread and roll the ball. The jumper can ask the others to vary the speed or keep it the same, according to ability. You can use balls of different sizes, and children change roles after 45 seconds.

Cigarette pack

This game is like smoking cigarettes. The more you smoke, the more difficulty you have being active. Designate an area of gym or playground as playing area. Select one person to be the cigarette, who chases others and tags them. The tagged players hook elbows or join hands and continue chasing others. The "cigarette chain" grows and grows. As it does, it has more difficulty moving. Split into two after chain reaches six players.

Partner cruise

Begin the activity with the students walking in a scatter formation around the gym. On command, have each student find a partner to face and shake their hand. This person is designated their "Handshake" partner. Again, the students scatter throughout the gym. On command, they must find their Handshake partners and shake hands. They then find a second partner and create a different handshake. The activity continues with students finding different partners and doing a different action with each partner, such as Back to Back, High Five, Sole Shake, and so on. Between partners, students walk or jog.

Over and under

Students find a partner. One partner makes a bridge on the floor while the other moves over, under, and around the bridge. This continues until you give a signal to switch, which notifies them to change positions. Try different types of bridges and movements.

Bean bag boogie

Each student has a bean bag placed on their head. Students move around the gym trying to keep the bean bag on their heads. If the student loses the bag, they freeze and another student has to come and pick it up for them.

Circle tag

Set up two concentric circles. Organize children into a large circle, with 10 feet between each child. With chalk, mark a circle for children to run around. Each child tries to tag the next child ahead in the circle. Tagged children move to an inside circle (marked in chalk) and run counterclockwise trying to tag the person in front of them. Children who are tagged on the inside circle move to the outside circle, changing directions as they switch circles.

Listen and move

Give the following instructions as quickly as the children can complete the tasks: run 20 steps to the left, skip 10 steps forward, jump as high as you can 10 times, make 5 big arm circles, gallop 20 steps forward, hop on the left foot 5 times, hop on the right foot 5 times.

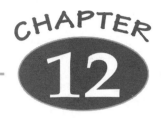

CHAPTER

12

Cool-Down Activities

Select cool-downs that allow an easy transition. For example, if children are already in pairs, the Meeting and Parting cool-down may be appropriate.

Rhythm run

Students form pairs and jog side by side around a baseball diamond or basketball court. Instruct them to run so their left and right feet move in rhythm together. When they can do this in pairs, have them progress to groups of four. Encourage students to remind their running partner to use good running techniques (see lesson 3). Slowly, change from jogging to walking.

Slo-mo skip

Set up four cones in square (40 × 40 yards). Students start by skipping one circuit at a fast rate, and each circuit thereafter slow down a little until they are in slo-mo.

Birthday line

Tell the students that they can no longer talk. The group challenge is to see how effectively the class can arrange themselves in order of birthdays from January 1 at one end to December 31 at the other end. They can use sign language but cannot talk. Have them complete some stretches when they are in line.

Leader cruise

Use a rectangular area marked by cones. Line up the class in two lines side by side. The entire class starts with a jog. The two students at the end jog to the front. As soon as the new leaders are in front, the next two jog to the front. Progressively, the lines slow down until they are walking.

Meeting and parting

Start with a partner in a specific place in the playing area. Jog side by side, moving apart from each other (for 10–12 yards) and then meeting again. Maintain eye contact with each other. Watch for others. Start by jogging; then slowly reduce pace to a fast walk, then a slower walk.

Body shapes

Students make their bodies into specific shapes, for example, narrow, round, twisted, crooked, small, flat, pointed, wide, curled. Start by having children move quickly from one shape to another; then slow down and ask children to move as slowly as possible.

Running shapes

Make sure students know circle, square, triangle, and rectangle shapes. Tell them to run in a specific area and make one of the shapes with their run.

Gradually, reduce the speed of the run until they are walking. Shapes can be a large or small. Call out a designated shape.

Statue run

Students run and on a signal assume a statue pose a few seconds before jogging again.

Alphabet circle

Students stand in a circle. Give each student a letter. Spell a word out loud and student squats down.

Team train

In groups of four or five, students stand in single file, holding onto the waist of the person in front. The leader moves the train around the play area. Change leaders. Trains begin to move slower as the cool-down continues.

Agility run

In playing area put out cones, and students have to weave in and out of them, careful not to collide with each other. Emphasize weaving patterns. Slow down as cool-down continues.

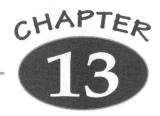

Exercises

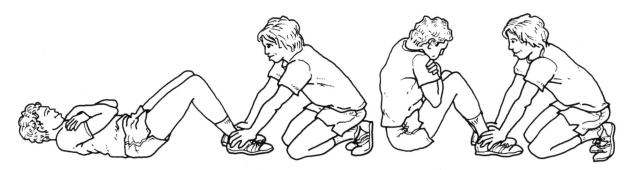

Sit-ups. Lie on back with knees bent (12–18 inch gap between feet and buttocks) and arms across chest. Lift upper body toward knees until arms touch thighs and lower until midback touches floor.

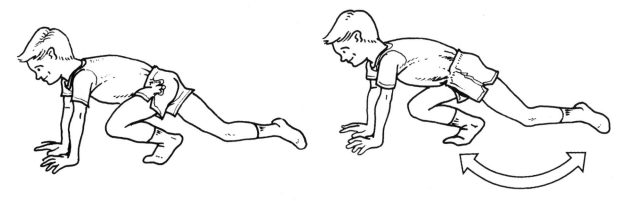

Mountain climbers. In front support position, bring the right knee up under chest and extend the left leg backward. Quickly switch leg positions, keeping a rhythmic movement pattern.

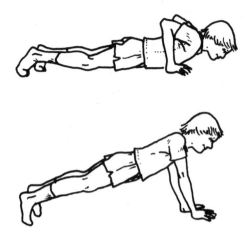

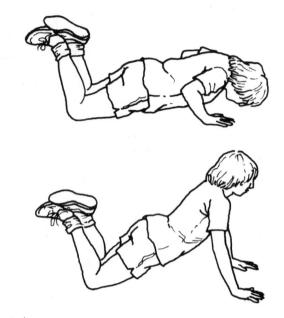

Push-ups.   Lie on stomach with chest touching floor and feet together. Hands are under the shoulders. Push and raise body by extending arms. Raise body in straight line, not allowing back to sway. Lower body until chin touches ground.

Modified push-ups.   Do as regular push-ups, only push up from knees, not feet.

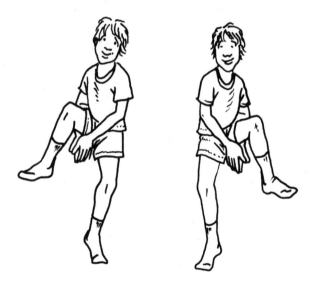

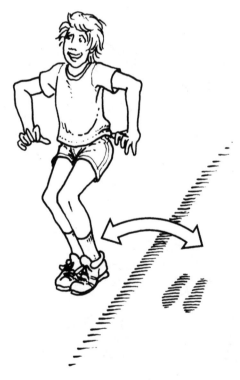

Clappers.   Hop on left foot, kick the right leg up, and clap your hands under the right leg. Hop on the right foot, kick the left leg up, and clap your hands under it. Land on the ball of the foot each time.

Skier.   With both feet together, jump from side to side over a line or jump rope.

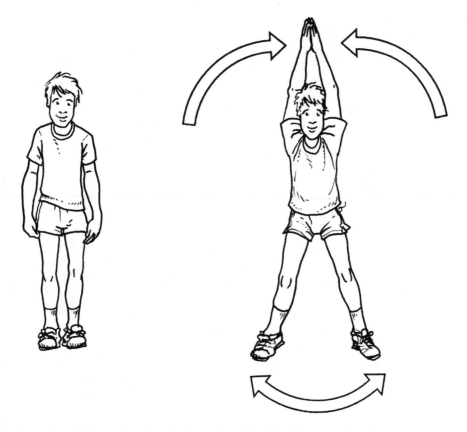

Jumping jacks.   Stand with arms by sides. Simultaneously raise arms above head and move legs shoulder-width apart. Then bring arms to sides and feet together.

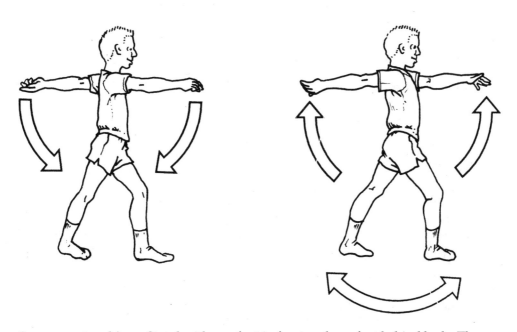

Cross-country skier.   Stand with one foot in front and one foot behind body. The opposite arm is also in front of the body. Jump and change positions of feet and arms.

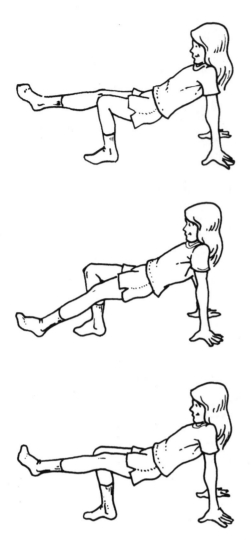

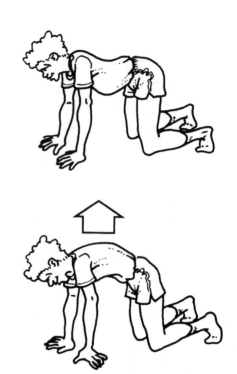

Bridge back.   On hands and knees in a crawling position, contract abdominal muscles and arch back as high as possible. Return to starting position.

Crab legs.   Support weight on hands and feet. Alternatively kick legs out away from body. Each kick counts as one repetition.

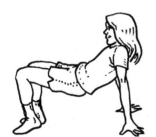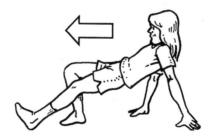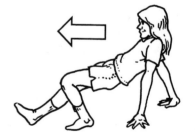

Crab walker.   From sitting position, push body off the ground and support weight on hands and feet. Move body forward three steps and backward three steps.

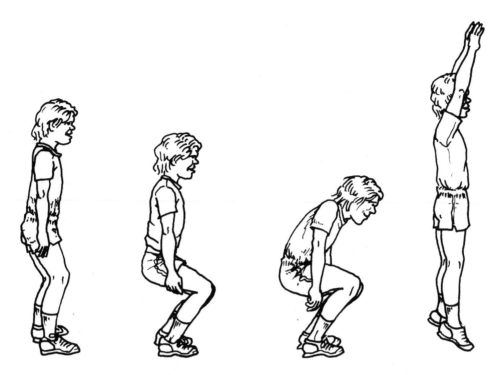

Jack-in-the-box.   Squat down low and pretend you are hiding in a box. Spring up reaching as high as you can. Return to starting position.

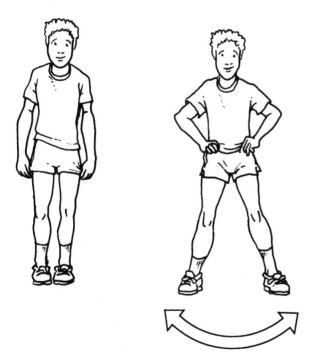

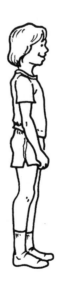

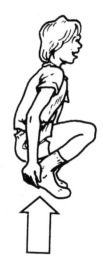

Heel touches.   Stand in an upright position with feet shoulder-width apart and arms fully extended at the sides. Jump vertically and touch the heels with the hands as the knees move to the chest.

Stride jumps.   Stand with feet together. Jump off ground so feet are spread three feet apart. Return to starting position.

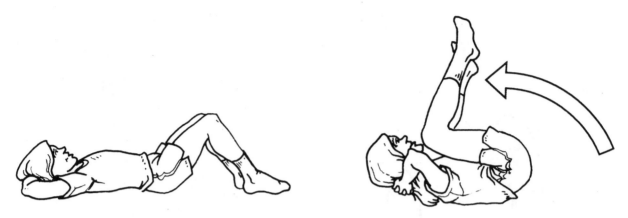

Reverse sit-ups.   Lie on back with legs together and knees bent. Bend at the waist and bring knees to chest. Lower legs to starting position.

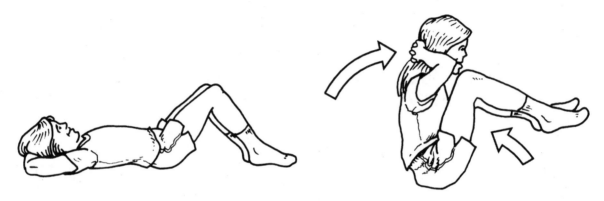

Crunches.   Lie on back with legs together and legs and knees bent, forming a 90-degree angle. Hands are behind head. Bring knees and elbows together, directly over waist area. Return to starting position.

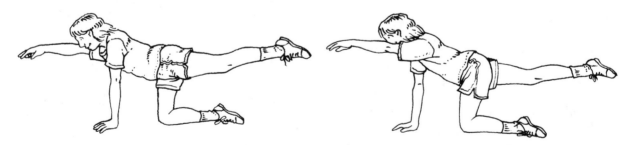

Cross body lift.   Assume an all fours position with your hands on the floor directly under your shoulders. In this position, raise one arm and the opposite leg simultaneously until they are slightly higher than your back. Then lower both simultaneously. Repeat this action with the opposite arm and leg in alternating fashion.

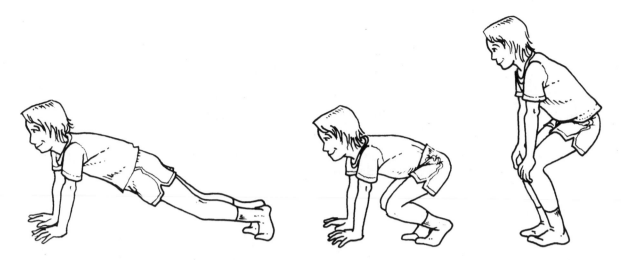

Squat thrusts.   In push-up position quickly move legs toward hands and jump high into the air.

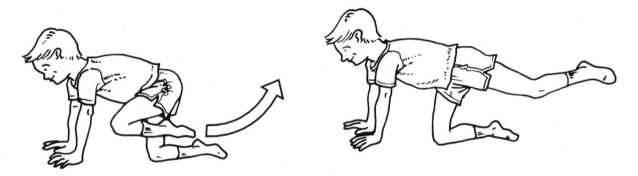

Leg extensions.   On all fours with legs square and right knee bent, raise right leg to side. Extend your leg forward and backward, parallel to the floor, then lower to the ground. Move legs only and keep upper body still. Change legs.

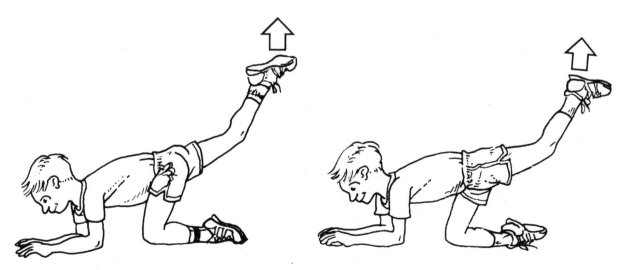

Skyscrapers.   Kneel on all fours. Lower weight to forearms and tighten abdominal muscles. Raise bent leg behind and push it to the ceiling. Flex and point the foot.

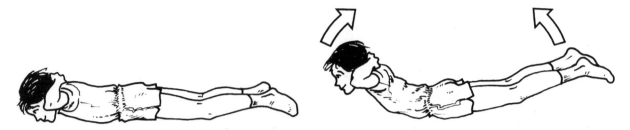

Chest raises.   Lie on stomach with feet together and hands clasped behind head. Raise head and chest away from ground and slowly lower to starting position.

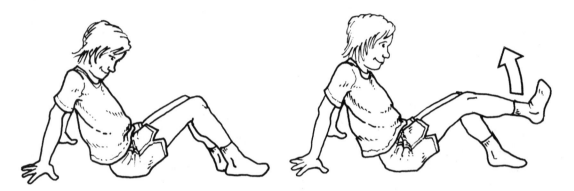

Thigh lifts.   Begin in the half-hook, half-long sit position. Raise and lower the extended leg. Change leg and raise.

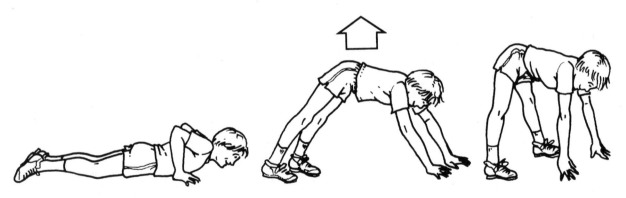

Inchworm.   Lie on stomach. Keep hands still and take small steps forward toward your hands. Then move feet back away from hands to the lying position.

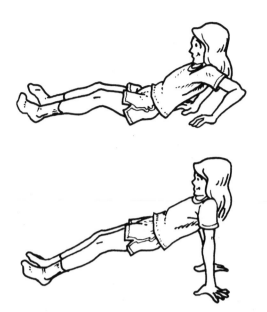

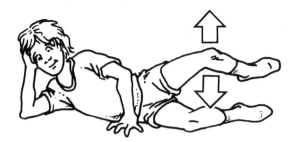

Side leg raises.   Lie on your right side with your head resting on your right hand and your left hand flat on the mat in front of you for support. Raise your upper leg. Repeat, changing sides.

Reverse push-ups.   In back support position, bend elbows to slowly lower body to the floor. Straighten elbows to raise body away from floor.

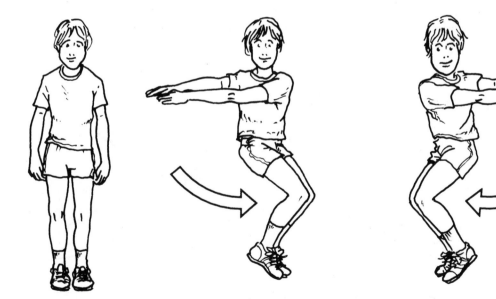

Jump twisters.   Stand with feet together, knees slightly bent. Thrust both arms to right while moving legs (from waist) to the left. Reverse action with arms moving to the left and legs to the right.

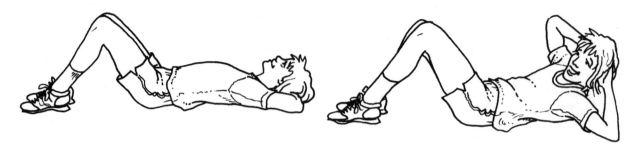

Obliques.   Lie on back with knees bent, feet on floor with hands held lightly behind head. Lift shoulder and upper torso off the floor twisting one elbow toward opposite knee. Do not pull head and neck with hands. Return to starting position and repeat on other side. Press spine to floor so hips do not roll.

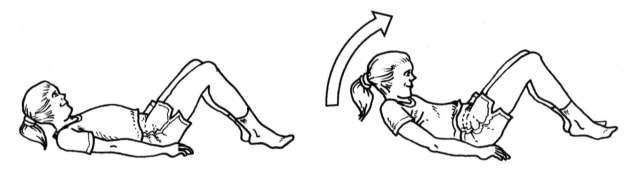

Curl-ups.   Lie on back with knees at a 90-degree angle and arms extended by side. Lift head until upper back is raised from floor and the chin touches the chest. Return to floor.

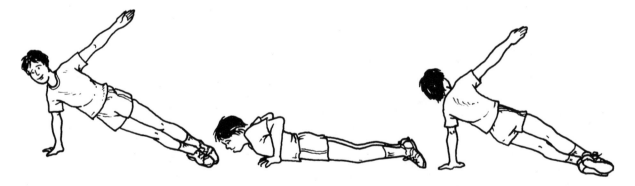

Side standers.   Lie on stomach with chest touching floor. Raise body in push-up fashion and rotate body so you support weight on right hand and foot. Return to starting position and support weight on left hand and foot.

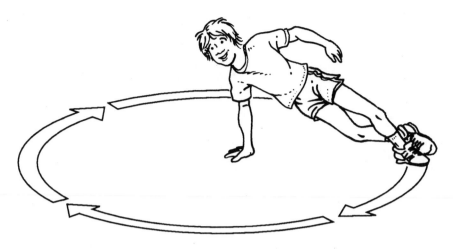

Coffee grinder.   Pivot on a supporting hand. Work feet around hand making a complete circle while keeping the body straight.

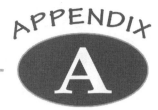

APPENDIX A

Physical Fitness Testing

Physical fitness testing has traditionally been a part of physical education. We believe this should continue, but with the following concepts clearly in mind:

- Teach children to test themselves. Children who learn to test themselves will know their current fitness levels and develop skills to use in later life.
- Self-evaluation, rather than comparison to others is important. Heredity, maturity, and age have much to do with fitness performance. Use test results to help students plan personal fitness programs.
- Explain why fitness testing is important. Reaching acceptable health fitness standards provided by programs, helping children identify their own strengths and weaknesses, and allowing children to monitor their improvement are all good reasons for physical fitness testing.
- If you are going to use awards, clearly explain the procedure for receiving awards. Use an incentive program that rewards participation and effort.

The following physical fitness test programs are available:

Physical Best
American Alliance for Health, Physical
Education, Recreation and Dance
1900 Association Drive
Reston, VA 22091.

President's Challenge
President's Council on Physical Fitness
and Sports
450 Fifth Street NW, Room 7103
Washington, DC 20001.

Physical Fitness Program
Amateur Athletic Union
Poplars Building
Bloomington, IN 47405.

Fitnessgram
Institute for Aerobic Fitness Research
12330 Preston Road
Dallas, TX 74230
1-800-635-7050.

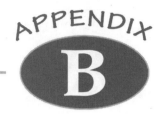

APPENDIX B

Parent Letter

You may use this sample letter as a guide for informing parents of the program and soliciting their involvement, or you may want to develop your own format. The goal for the program is to improve attitudes toward fitness in both students and parents, and to increase communication between the home and school.

Dear Parents:

Your child will be participating in a new physical fitness program soon. The name of the program is Health-Related Fitness. It will begin on (date) and run approximately _____ weeks.

In this program, we will explore a variety of topics related to health, physical fitness, and nutrition. We will emphasize establishing healthy habits that will last a lifetime. Students will learn how to assess their individual fitness level based on the knowledge they gain in this program and will be able to design their personal fitness program. They will learn how to maintain a healthy level of physical fitness. Also, they will learn about heart-healthy nutrition and how to improve their eating habits.

Your child will be involved in a wide range of fitness and nutrition activities. The weekly schedule is three days of physical activity and two days of classroom instruction. Students will be expected to perform only at their own level. Our goal is to help each student strive for and recognize individual gains in his or her fitness level.

If you have questions or would like further information about this program, please contact me by phone or letter. You will be receiving information about Family Fitness activities. We hope you will be able to participate and enjoy the fun with your children. We hope you can give support and encouragement to your child for continued improvement in health and fitness.

Please call me if you have any questions.

Sincerely,

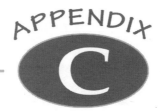

APPENDIX
C

Additional Resources

Bennett, J.P., and A. Kamiya. 1986. *Fitness and fun for everyone.* Durham, NC: Great Activities.

Cames, C. 1983. *Awesome elementary school physical education activities.* Carmichael, CA: Education.

Corbin, C.B., and R.P. Pangrazi. 1990. *Teaching strategies for improving youth fitness.* Dallas: Institute for Aerobics Research.

Foster, E.R., K. Hartinger, and K.A. Smith. 1992. *Fitness fun.* Champaign, IL: Human Kinetics.

Hopper, C. 1988. *The sports confident child.* New York: Pantheon Books.

Landy, J.M., and M.L. Landy. 1992. *Ready-to-use P.E. activities for grades K-2.* West Nyack, NY: Parker.

Pangrazi, R.P., and V.P. Dauer. 1992. *Dynamic physical education for elementary school children.* New York: Macmillan.

Petray, C.K., and S.L. Blazer. 1987. *Health-related physical fitness.* Edina, MN: Burgess.

Stillwell, J.L., and J.R. Stockard. 1988. *More fitness activities for children.* Durham, NC: Great Activities.

Index

About the Authors

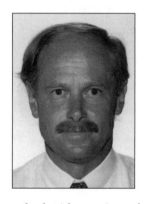

Chris Hopper, PhD, is department chair and professor of physical education at Humboldt State University in Arcata, California.

Hopper brings a variety of experiences in physical education to his writing. Since 1976 he has taught physical education at the elementary through college level. He also has consulted with a variety of organizations, including the United States Department of Education, the Boys Clubs of America, and the American Sport Education Program. Throughout his career he has coached both youth and collegiate soccer, serving as head coach of men's soccer at Humboldt State University.

In 1982 Hopper earned his PhD in physical education from the University of Oregon. Much of his research has focused on improving children's physical fitness and nutrition. He has published numerous articles in the *Journal of Physical Education, Recreation and Dance; Scholastic Coach; Adapted Physical Activity Quarterly;* and the *Research Quarterly for Exercise and Sport.* He is coauthor of *Coaching Soccer Effectively* and author of *The Sports-Confident Child.*

Hopper is a member of the American Alliance for Health, Physical Education, Recreation and Dance, the National Consortium on Physical Education and Recreation for Individuals With Disabilities; and the American Council on Rural Special Education.

Hopper, who lives in Ferndale, California, with his wife, Renee, and their three children, enjoys soccer, golf, and waterskiing.

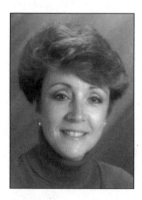

Kathy D. Munoz, EdD, is assistant professor in the Department of Health and Physical Education at Humboldt State University.

Munoz has a master's in food and nutrition from Oregon State University and an EdD in education and curriculum design from the University of Southern California. As a registered dietitian and home economics teacher, she has taught nutrition to a wide variety of ages and backgrounds, including secondary, community college, and university students. She also worked with students, athletes, and community members as a counselor at the Eating Disorder Clinic in Humboldt.

In 1989 Munoz won the Meritorious Performance and Professional Promise Award from Humboldt State for teaching nutrition. She is advisor to the Youth Education Services (YES) Nutrition for Kids program, a role she filled also for the Student Home Economics Association.

A member of the American Dietetic Association, American College of Nutrition, and the Society for Nutrition Education, Munoz lives in Fortuna, California, with her husband, Richard, and their three children. She pursues outdoor sports, reading, and traveling in her spare time.

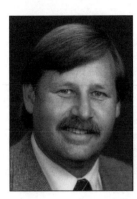

Bruce Fisher has received several honors for teaching excellence, including 1991 California Teacher of the Year, 1991 Professional Best Award, and the ABC-TV Favorite Teacher Award. A classroom teacher since 1975, he has created meaningful activities and lessons to teach fitness and nutrition to students at all grade levels.

As a member of the California State Department of Education's Health and Physical Education committee since 1991, Fisher helped design and develop the health and physical education frameworks for California. He has served on educational and curriculum development committees throughout his career, including the Family Wellness Project, and he also has presented at education conferences across the country.

In 1991 Fisher wrote the feature article for *Learning Magazine* on health and nutrition. Now with the Jet Propulsion Lab, Johns Hopkins University, and San Diego State University, he is writing the curriculum for NASA's KidSat/Project YES.

Fisher lives in Fieldbrook, California, with his wife, Mindi, and their daughter, Jenny. His hobbies include aviation, aerospace, astronomy, and photography.

Integrate health and fitness lessons into your curriculum with these ready-to-use activities

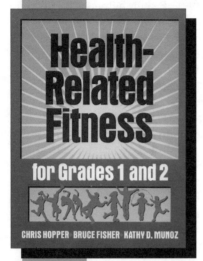

1996 • Paper • 128 pp
Item BHOP0498
ISBN 0-87322-498-1
$16.00 ($23.95 Canadian)

1996 • Paper • 136 pp
Item BHOP0499
ISBN 0-87322-499-X
$16.00 ($23.95 Canadian)

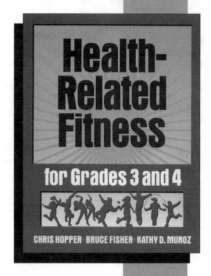

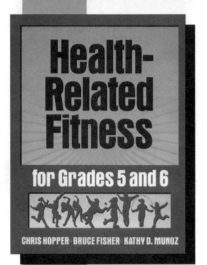

1996 • Paper • Approx 160 pp
Item BHOP0480
ISBN 0-88011-480-0
$18.00 ($26.95 Canadian)

Each *Health-Related Fitness* book provides 45 grade-appropriate, cross-curricular lessons and activities in physical fitness and nutrition. The classroom-tested programs in each book provide nine weeks of plans for five 30-minute, ready-to-use lessons.

This unique, hands-on curriculum includes homework assignments with family activities, cooperative learning experiences, cross-curricular activities to stimulate critical thinking skills, reproducible handouts, easy-to-understand adaptable scripts, activities based on state and national health standards, and lessons that require either no equipment or simple materials readily available.

Part I of each book outlines lessons on cardiovascular fitness, strength, endurance, flexibility, and nutrition to help you prepare students for a healthy lifestyle. **Part II** describes the different kinds of elements you should teach in each lesson, including stretches, warm-ups, cool-downs, and exercises.

Human Kinetics
The Information Leader in Physical Activity
http://www.humankinetics.com/

2335

Prices are subject to change.

M8133-In
85